NATIONAL ACADEMIES *Sciences Engineering Medicine*

NATIONAL ACADEMIES PRESS
Washington, DC

Exploring Psyc and Entactoge as Treatments for Psychiatric Disorders

Lisa Bain, Chanel Matney,
Sheena M. Posey Norris, and
Clare Stroud, *Rapporteurs*

Forum on Neuroscience and
Nervous System Disorders

Board on Health Sciences Policy

Health and Medicine Division

Proceedings of a Workshop

THE NATIONAL ACADEMIES PRESS 500 Fifth Street, NW Washington, DC 20001

This activity was supported by contracts between the National Academy of Sciences and the Alzheimer's Association; California Institute for Regenerative Medicine; Cerevel Therapeutics; Cohen Veterans Bioscience; Department of Health and Human Services' Food and Drug Administration (R13FD005362) and National Institutes of Health (NIH) (75N98019F00769 [Under Master Base HHSN263201800029I]) through the National Center for Complementary and Integrative Health, National Eye Institute, National Institute of Environmental Health Sciences, National Institute of Mental Health, National Institute of Neurological Disorders and Stroke, National Institute on Aging, National Institute on Alcohol Abuse and Alcoholism, National Institute on Drug Abuse, and NIH BRAIN Initiative; Department of Veterans Affairs (36C24E20C0009); Eisai Inc.; Eli Lilly and Company; Foundation for the National Institutes of Health; Gatsby Charitable Foundation; Janssen Research & Development, LLC; Karuna Therapeutics; Lundbeck Research USA; Merck Research Laboratories; The Michael J. Fox Foundation for Parkinson's Research; National Multiple Sclerosis Society; National Science Foundation (DBI-1839674); One Mind; Simons Foundation Autism Research Initiative; Takeda Pharmaceuticals International, Inc.; and Wellcome Trust. Any opinions, findings, conclusions, or recommendations expressed in this publication do not necessarily reflect the views of any organization or agency that provided support for the project.

International Standard Book Number-13: 978-0-309-69137-6
International Standard Book Number-10: 0-309-69137-0
Digital Object Identifier: https://doi.org/10.17226/26648

This publication is available from the National Academies Press, 500 Fifth Street, NW, Keck 360, Washington, DC 20001; (800) 624-6242 or (202) 334-3313; http://www.nap.edu.

Printed in the United States of America.

Suggested citation: National Academies of Sciences, Engineering, and Medicine. 2022. *Exploring psychedelics and entactogens as treatments for psychiatric disorders: Proceedings of a workshop.* Washington, DC: The National Academies Press. https://doi.org/10.17226/26648.

The **National Academy of Sciences** was established in 1863 by an Act of Congress, signed by President Lincoln, as a private, nongovernmental institution to advise the nation on issues related to science and technology. Members are elected by their peers for outstanding contributions to research. Dr. Marcia McNutt is president.

The **National Academy of Engineering** was established in 1964 under the charter of the National Academy of Sciences to bring the practices of engineering to advising the nation. Members are elected by their peers for extraordinary contributions to engineering. Dr. John L. Anderson is president.

The **National Academy of Medicine** (formerly the Institute of Medicine) was established in 1970 under the charter of the National Academy of Sciences to advise the nation on medical and health issues. Members are elected by their peers for distinguished contributions to medicine and health. Dr. Victor J. Dzau is president.

The three Academies work together as the **National Academies of Sciences, Engineering, and Medicine** to provide independent, objective analysis and advice to the nation and conduct other activities to solve complex problems and inform public policy decisions. The National Academies also encourage education and research, recognize outstanding contributions to knowledge, and increase public understanding in matters of science, engineering, and medicine.

Learn more about the National Academies of Sciences, Engineering, and Medicine at **www.nationalacademies.org**.

Consensus Study Reports published by the National Academies of Sciences, Engineering, and Medicine document the evidence-based consensus on the study's statement of task by an authoring committee of experts. Reports typically include findings, conclusions, and recommendations based on information gathered by the committee and the committee's deliberations. Each report has been subjected to a rigorous and independent peer-review process and it represents the position of the National Academies on the statement of task.

Proceedings published by the National Academies of Sciences, Engineering, and Medicine chronicle the presentations and discussions at a workshop, symposium, or other event convened by the National Academies. The statements and opinions contained in proceedings are those of the participants and are not endorsed by other participants, the planning committee, or the National Academies.

Rapid Expert Consultations published by the National Academies of Sciences, Engineering, and Medicine are authored by subject-matter experts on narrowly focused topics that can be supported by a body of evidence. The discussions contained in rapid expert consultations are considered those of the authors and do not contain policy recommendations. Rapid expert consultations are reviewed by the institution before release.

For information about other products and activities of the National Academies, please visit www.nationalacademies.org/about/whatwedo.

EXPLORING PSYCHEDELICS AND ENTACTOGENS AS TREATMENTS FOR PSYCHIATRIC DISORDERS[1]

SARAH H. LISANBY (*Co-Chair*), National Institute of Mental Health
GERARD SANACORA (*Co-Chair*), Yale University
PAUL APPELBAUM, Columbia University
CHARMA DUDLEY, National Alliance on Mental Illness
ALLYSON GAGE, Cohen Veterans Bioscience
JAVIER GONZALEZ-MAÉSO, Virginia Commonwealth University
ROLAND GRIFFITHS, Johns Hopkins University
VICTORIA HALE, Sacred Medicines
JOHN KRYSTAL, Yale University
TRISTAN McCLURE-BEGLEY, Defense Advanced Research Projects Agency
JAVIER MUÑIZ, Food and Drug Administration
SRINIVAS RAO, atai Life Sciences
RITA VALENTINO, National Institute on Drug Abuse

Health and Medicine Division Staff

CHANEL MATNEY, Program Officer
EDEN NELEMAN, Senior Program Assistant
SHEENA M. POSEY NORRIS, Director, Forum on Neuroscience and Nervous System Disorders
CLARE STROUD, Senior Board Director, Board on Health Sciences Policy

---

[1] The National Academies of Sciences, Engineering, and Medicine's planning committees are solely responsible for organizing the workshop, identifying topics, and choosing speakers. The responsibility for the published Proceedings of a Workshop rests with the workshop rapporteurs and the institution.

FORUM ON NEUROSCIENCE AND NERVOUS SYSTEM DISORDERS[1]

FRANCES JENSEN (*Co-Chair*), University of Pennsylvania
JOHN KRYSTAL (*Co-Chair*), Yale University
SUSAN AMARA, National Institute of Mental Health
ELINE APPELMANS, Foundation for the National Institutes of Health
KATJA BROSE, Chan Zuckerberg Initiative
EMERY BROWN, Harvard Medical School and Massachusetts Institute of Technology
JOSEPH BUXBAUM, Icahn School of Medicine at Mount Sinai
SARAH CADDICK, Gatsby Charitable Foundation
ROSA CANET-AVILÉS, California Institute for Regenerative Medicine
MARIA CARRILLO, Alzheimer's Association
EDWARD CHANG, University of California, San Francisco (*until July 2022*)
MICHAEL CHIANG, National Eye Institute
TIMOTHY COETZEE, National Multiple Sclerosis Society
JONATHAN COHEN, Princeton University
BEVERLY DAVIDSON, University of Pennsylvania (*from August 2022*)
BILLY DUNN, Food and Drug Administration
MICHAEL EGAN, Merck Research Laboratories
MICHELLE ELEKONICH, National Science Foundation
NITA FARAHANY, Duke University
EVA FELDMAN, University of Michigan (*from August 2022*)
BRIAN FISKE, The Michael J. Fox Foundation for Parkinson's Research
JOSHUA A. GORDON, National Institute of Mental Health
MAGALI HAAS, Cohen Veterans Bioscience
RICHARD HODES, National Institute on Aging
STUART HOFFMAN, Department of Veterans Affairs
YASMIN HURD, Icahn School of Medicine at Mount Sinai
STEVEN HYMAN, Broad Institute of Massachusetts Institute of Technology and Harvard University
MICHAEL IRIZARRY, Eisai Inc.
PUSHKAR JOSHI, One Mind
GEORGE KOOB, National Institute on Alcohol Abuse and Alcoholism
WALTER KOROSHETZ, National Institute of Neurological Disorders and Stroke
HUSSEINI MANJI, Johnson & Johnson (*until June 2022*)
BILL MARTIN, Johnson & Johnson (*from July 2022*)

---

[1] The National Academies of Sciences, Engineering, and Medicine's forums and roundtables do not issue, review, or approve individual documents. The responsibility for the published *Proceedings of a Workshop* rests with the workshop rapporteurs and the institution.

Reviewers

This Proceedings of a Workshop was reviewed in draft form by individuals chosen for their diverse perspectives and technical expertise. The purpose of this independent review is to provide candid and critical comments that will assist the National Academies of Sciences, Engineering, and Medicine in making each published proceedings as sound as possible and to ensure that it meets the institutional standards for quality, objectivity, evidence, and responsiveness to the charge. The review comments and draft manuscript remain confidential to protect the integrity of the process.

We thank the following individuals for their review of this proceedings:

PAUL APPELBAUM, Columbia University
GÜL DÖLEN, Johns Hopkins University
CAROLINE DORSEN, Rutgers University School of Nursing
WALTER DUNN, University of California, Los Angeles
KATRIN PRELLER, University of Zurich
CARLOS ZARATE, The George Washington University

Although the reviewers listed above provided many constructive comments and suggestions, they were not asked to endorse the content of the proceedings nor did they see the final draft before its release. The review of this proceedings was overseen by **LESLIE Z. BENET,** University of California, San Francisco. He was responsible for making certain that an independent examination of this proceedings was carried out in accordance with standards of the National Academies and that all review comments were carefully considered. Responsibility for the final content rests entirely with the rapporteurs and the National Academies.

Contents

Acronyms and Abbreviations

$5\text{-}HT_{1A}$	Serotonin 1A receptor
$5\text{-}HT_{2A}$	Serotonin 2A receptor
ACE	Accept, Connect, Embody
ACT	Acceptance Commitment Therapy
AMPA	α-amino-3-hydroxy-5-methyl-4-isoxazole propionic acid
BDNF	brain derived neurotrophic factor
CAPS-IV	Clinician-Administered PTSD Scale for DSM-IV
CPT	Current Procedural Terminology
DARPA	Defense Advanced Research Projects Agency
DEA	Drug Enforcement Administration
DMT	dimethyl tryptamine
DOI	1-(2,5-dimethoxy-4-iodophenyl)-2-aminopropane
DSM	*Diagnostic and Statistical Manual of Mental Disorders*
FDA	Food and Drug Administration
fMRI	functional magnetic resonance imagining
GABA	Gamma-Amniobutyric Acid
GMP	Good Manufacturing Practice

LGBTQIA+	lesbian, gay, bisexual, transgender, queer, intersex, asexual
LSD	lysergic acid diethylamide
MADRS	Montgomery-Åsperg Depression Rating Scale
MAPS	Multidisciplinary Association for Psychedelic Studies
MDMA	3,4-Methylenedioxymethamphetamine
mPFC	medial prefrontal cortex
MRI	magnetic resonance imaging
mTOR	mammalian/mechanistic target of rapamycin
NAMI	National Alliance on Mental Illness
NDA	New Drug Application
NIDA	National Institute on Drug Abuse
NIH	National Institutes of Health
NIMH	National Institute of Mental Health
OCD	obsessive-compulsive disorder
PBC	public benefit corporation
PCP	phencyclidine
PET	positron emission tomography
PFC	prefrontal cortex
PTSD	posttraumatic stress disorder
REMS	risk evaluation and mitigation strategy
RTN	reticular thalamic nuclei
SAMHSA	Substance Abuse and Mental Health Services Administration
SNRI	selective noradrenaline reuptake inhibitor
SSRI	selective serotonin reuptake inhibitor
SV2A	synaptic vesicle protein 2A
TBG	tabernanthalog
TRD	treatment-resistant depression
trkB	tyrosine protein kinase B
VA	Department of Veterans Affairs
VEH	vehicle control

1

Introduction and Background[1]

Psychiatric illnesses—such as major depressive disorder, anxiety disorder, substance use disorder, and posttraumatic stress disorder (PTSD)—are widely prevalent and represent a substantial health burden worldwide (GBD 2019 Mental Disorders Collaborators, 2022). According to the National Alliance on Mental Illness (NAMI), nearly one in five Americans live with a diagnosed mental illness.[2] Yet, conventional medications for mental illnesses often fail to relieve patients of disruptive and disabling symptoms.

It has long been known that the classic psychedelics (namely, lysergic acid diethylamide [LSD] and psilocybin) and entactogens (namely, 3,4-methylenedioxymethamphetamine [MDMA])[3] can facilitate profound and

---

[1] The planning committee's role was limited to planning the workshop, and the Proceedings of a Workshop was prepared by the workshop rapporteurs as a factual summary of what occurred at the workshop. Statements, recommendations, and opinions expressed are those of individual presenters and participants; have not been endorsed or verified by the Health and Medicine Division of the National Academies of Sciences, Engineering, and Medicine; and should not be construed as reflecting any group consensus.

[2] To learn more about the prevalence of mental illness and the National Alliance on Mental Illness, see https://www.nami.org/mhstats (accessed June 12, 2022).

[3] In these proceedings, the term "psychedelics" refers to hallucination-inducing drugs with a mechanism of action that is thought to be primarily mediated through 5HT receptor agonism. These so-called serotonergic hallucinogens induce an altered state of consciousness characterized by profound alterations in mood, thought process, and perception (De Gregorio et al., 2021a; Vollenweider and Kometer, 2010). This pharmacological category is also referred to as the "classic psychedelics." The term "entactogens" (sometimes referred to as "empathogens," but with "entactogens" predominating in usage) refers to a pharmacological class of drug that induces feelings of empathy, connectedness, and well-being through a

persistent changes in cognitive, sensory, and psychoemotional states (Rucker et al., 2022). However, existing and emerging evidence suggesting that these substances may also be useful as tools to alleviate mental illness has sparked a renaissance of interest by investigators, clinicians, drug developers, and patient advocates in recent years. In response to this renewed interest, the National Academies of Sciences, Engineering, and Medicine's Forum on Neuroscience and Nervous System Disorders (Neuroscience Forum) convened a workshop on March 29 and 30, 2022, to explore the use of psychedelics and entactogens as treatments for psychiatric disorders.[4]

"There's such tremendous excitement about these agents and their potential to represent a paradigm shift in psychiatric therapeutics, in which we have the hope of rapidly acting and long-lasting treatments," said Sarah H. "Holly" Lisanby, director of translational research at the National Institute of Mental Health (NIMH), and professor emeritus of psychiatry at Duke University.

While optimism about the use of psychedelics and entactogens is warranted by the data available, Gerard Sanacora, Gross Professor of Psychiatry at the Yale University School of Medicine and workshop co-chair, said this optimism must be balanced with concerns about the complexity, ethics, licensing, regulatory oversight, public health, and health equity. "We still have a long way to go," he said, cautioning against letting the excitement surrounding potential clinical benefits get too far ahead of actual clinical efficacy and safety data. He added that the anecdotal reports of clinical benefit and the limited clinical trials that have been completed have "spurred a tremendous [number] of back-translational efforts to further understand the potential mechanisms of action."

THE NATIONAL INSTITUTES OF HEALTH EXAMINES RESEARCH OPPORTUNITIES AND GAPS

A surge in scientific and public interest in the therapeutic potential of psychedelics prompted the National Institutes of Health (NIH) to convene a workshop[5] in January 2022 to examine the challenges, opportunities, and research gaps that need to be addressed to advance this therapeutic

---

mechanism of action involving carrier-mediated serotonin release from neuronal stores. This drug class includes 3,4-methylenedioxymethamphetamine (MDMA) and other substances with a similar psychopharmacological effect (Kyzar et al., 2017; Vollenweider, 2001).

[4] To learn more about the workshop, go to https://www.nationalacademies.org/event/03-29-2022/exploring-psychedelics-and-entactogens-as-treatments-for-psychiatric-disorders-a-workshop (accessed June 22, 2022).

[5] For information on the NIH Workshop on Psychedelics as Therapeutics: Gaps, Challenges and Opportunities, see https://nida.nih.gov/news-events/meetings-events/2022/01/nih-workshop-psychedelics-therapeutics-gaps-challenges-opportunities (accessed July 6, 2022).

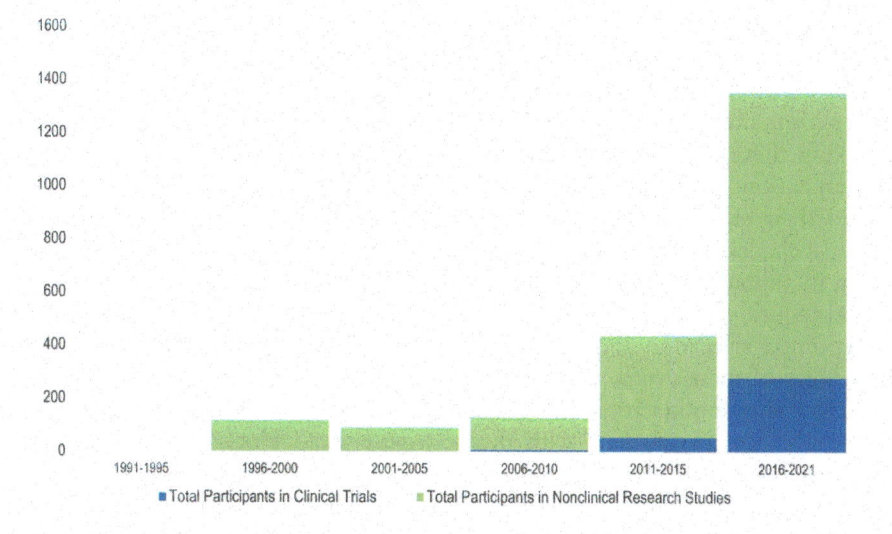

FIGURE 1-1 Psychedelics research 1991–2021. A summary of published research on the use of psychedelics for therapeutic purposes shows that the total number of participants in clinical trials (blue) and non-clinical research studies (green) has increased markedly over the past two decades.
SOURCES: Presented by Nora Volkow, March 29, 2022; Bender and Hellerstein, 2022.

paradigm, said Nora Volkow, director of the National Institute on Drug Abuse (NIDA). As shown in Figure 1-1, both clinical trials and non-clinical research studies have accelerated rapidly over the past two decades, particularly in the past 5 years. However, Volkow noted that most clinical trials have small sample sizes and are non-randomized.

Volkow added that the recreational use of hallucinogen-inducing drugs among college-age adults also increased between 2019 and 2020 (Schulenberg et al., 2021), which she attributed both to increased media attention and the stress of the COVID-19 pandemic.

The NIH workshop addressed the need for better categorization of psychedelic drugs,[6] including the classic psychedelics (namely, LSD and

---

[6] There are ongoing discussions in the field about when to use the term "psychedelic." The designation has meant different things since coined in the late 1950s. In this 2022 NIH Workshop, "psychedelics" was used in an inclusive umbrella fashion to refer collectively to the classic psychedelics (e.g., LSD and psilocybin), dissociative anesthetics (e.g., ketamine and PCP), and entactogens (e.g., MDMA). In contrast, this workshop proceedings designates "psychedelics" as the classic psychedelics (serotonergic hallucinogenic drugs), and treats dissociative anesthetics and entactogens as distinct pharmacological categories with overlapping effects on behavior and mind. For more information, see https://www.nimh.nih.gov/news/events/2022/psychedelics-as-therapeutics-gaps-challenges-and-opportunities (accessed June 12, 2022).

psilocybin), dissociative anesthetics such as ketamine and phencyclidine (PCP or "angel dust"), and entactogens such as MDMA. Volkow suggested that clustering drugs according to their molecular targets and mechanisms of action, rather than by the highly variable subjective experiences of people taking these substances, will facilitate advances in research, clearer communication, and ultimately a shared understanding of psychedelic drugs and their effects, both positive and negative. The role of neuroplasticity in psychedelic therapy was discussed extensively at the workshop, including in animal models where neuroplasticity changes have been linked with therapeutic effects, enabling the ability to potentially tailor interventions to maximize effects. In addition, the apparent low toxicity and low addiction liability of these drugs, although not across all classes (e.g., Johnson et al., 2018), was another topic of discussion. Some of the drugs like ibogaine (a non-classical psychedelic with dissociative effects) block cardiac calcium channels in the heart, potentially leading to cardiotoxicity (Corkey, 2018). In addition, recreational MDMA use has been associated with subclinical heart valve disease (Droogmans et al., 2007). Although rare, in certain instances, recreational use of these drugs can lead to adverse outcomes like overdose or suicidality. As it relates to addiction liability, "they can lead to repeated misuse and negative consequences, but this is distinct from the enhanced motivational drive that you see with the classical addictive drugs," said Volkow.

Characteristics of psychedelics such as neuroplasticity changes, low toxicity, and addiction liability suggest potential therapeutic benefits for depression and several other psychiatric disorders, including PTSD, obsessive-compulsive disorder (OCD), anorexia, autism spectrum disorder in adults, and substance use disorders. However, Volkow noted that major knowledge gaps exist related to safety, efficacy, dosing regimens, and concomitant therapies. While some evidence suggests that a greater mystical experience during psychedelics therapy correlates with higher efficacy (e.g., Griffiths et al., 2016), further investigation is needed, she said.

Sessions at the NIH workshop also focused on the challenges of conducting clinical trials and the need for objective surrogate outcome measures, as well as translation of the controlled conditions of psychedelic trials into real-world practice, said Volkow. Harmonized protocols for trials, including common inclusion criteria and methods for characterizing participants, are needed so that studies can be compared with one another, she said. Longer follow-up studies are needed to better understand long-term benefits and risks of psychedelic therapies. In addition, for therapies that demonstrate efficacy in clinical trials, a risk evaluation and mitigation strategy (REMS) will be needed to maximize the benefits and minimize the adverse effects of these therapies, said Volkow. Other outstanding questions discussed included who will pay for these trials and how to ensure that diverse populations have access to the research and any new treatments that emerge from it, she said.

WORKSHOP OBJECTIVES

The goals of this workshop are to follow up on the January 2022 NIH workshop to develop a deeper understanding of both the promise and the pitfalls of these agents, and the potential next steps that might be taken to realize their therapeutic potential, said Lisanby (see Box 1-1). The therapeutic benefits of ketamine, a dissociative anesthetic with psychedelic properties, was discussed in a prior National Academies workshop proceedings, and was therefore not addressed again here.[7]

ORGANIZATION OF THE PROCEEDINGS

Recognizing the ongoing debate in the field regarding nomenclature, for the purposes of this workshop and proceedings, "psychedelics" is used to refer to hallucination-inducing drugs with a mechanism of action that is thought to be primarily mediated through 5HT receptor agonism. These so-called serotonergic hallucinogens are substances that induce an altered state of consciousness that is characterized by profound alterations in mood, thought process, and perception (De Gregorio et al., 2021a; Vollenweider and Kometer, 2010). This pharmacological category is also referred to as the "classic psychedelics." The term "entactogens" (sometimes referred to as "empathogens," but with "entactogens" predominating in usage) refers to a pharmacological class of drug that induces feelings of empathy, connectedness, and well-being through a mechanism of action involving carrier-mediated serotonin release from neuronal stores. This drug class includes 3,4-methylenedioxymethamphetamine (MDMA) and other substances with a similar psychopharmacological effect (Kyzar et al., 2017; Vollenweider, 2001) psychoactive drugs that induce feelings of empathy and/or a desire for contact with others (Vollenweider, 2001).

Chapter 2 discusses the history of the use of psychedelics and entactogens (i.e., MDMA) for the treatment of psychiatric disorders from more than 7,000 years ago to the present time, including the personal experiences of two individuals who participated in clinical trials. Chapter 3 explores the varied mechanisms of action of the different classes of psychedelics and entactogens as well as key knowledge gaps, including the question of whether the subjective mystical experience is essential for a therapeutic

---

[7] To read those workshop proceedings, see https://nap.nationalacademies.org/catalog/26218/novel-molecular-targets-for-mood-disorders-and-psychosis-proceedings-of (accessed June 12, 2022).

BOX 1-1
Statement of Task

A planning committee of the National Academies of Sciences, Engineering, and Medicine will organize and conduct a 1.5-day virtual public workshop that brings together experts and key stakeholders from academia, government, industry, and non-profit organizations to explore the use of psychedelics and entactogens—including lysergic acid diethylamide (LSD), psilocybin, and 3,4-methylenedioxymethamphetamine (MDMA)—as treatments for psychiatric disorders, such as major depressive disorder, anxiety disorder, posttraumatic stress disorder, and substance use disorders.

Invited presentations and discussions will be designed to:

- Review the current state of knowledge regarding the mechanisms of action and pharmacokinetic/pharmacodynamic properties of these compounds, including considering the impact of polypharmacy;
- Discuss the current evidence on the clinical efficacy of psychedelics and entactogens to treat psychiatric conditions, including:
  o Exploring the role of adjunctive psychotherapy,
  o Whether hallucinogenic and dissociative side effects are essential to treatment efficacy, and
  o Clarifying the importance of psychosocial contexts;
- Consider the role of biomarkers to target treatments, stratify patients, and predict safety profiles;
- Explore appropriate clinical trial design, the need for standardization of treatment regimens, the challenge of blinding and accounting for placebo effects, and regulatory considerations;
- Discuss the impacts of these compounds' legal status and scheduling classifications on research;
- Explore questions of biomedical ethics such as those regarding patient protections and consent, standards of clinical training and quality assurance, off-label use, equitable access to treatment options, and engagement with public interest and experimentation; and
- Discuss open research questions, policy needs, and opportunities to move the field forward.

The planning committee will develop the agenda for the workshop, select and invite speakers and discussants, and moderate the discussions. A proceedings of the presentations and discussions at the workshop will be prepared by designated rapporteurs in accordance with institutional guidelines.

effect. The unique challenges for clinical development posed by these agents, as well as current clinical trial evidence for the efficacy of MDMA and psilocybin, are explored in Chapter 4. Considerations to ensure equitable access to psychedelic treatment are discussed in Chapter 5. Chapter 6 provides a summary of the workshop and the thoughts of leaders in the field regarding potential key themes to navigate the future of psychedelic treatment. References cited throughout this proceedings are listed in Appendix A, and the workshop agenda is in Appendix B.

During the workshop, public attendees were able to ask questions and submit comments via an online chat platform, which were later posed by session moderators in the open panel discussions. These discussions are captured throughout this proceedings.

2

History and Current Status of Psychedelics and Entactogens for the Treatment of Psychiatric Disorders

---

HIGHLIGHTS

- Psychedelic mushrooms have been used for shamanic and medicinal practices for more than 7,000 years, with the first Western report of their properties published in 1957 (Grob).
- The nomenclature around psychedelic compounds remains undefined despite many terms that have been proposed, including hallucinogen, entheogen, psychomimetic, mysticomimetic, and phantasticant (Grob).
- Clinical research on psychedelics expanded from the 1940s to the 1960s, but unraveled as the drugs seeped out of research settings and became associated with the counterculture (Grob).
- 3,4-Methylenedioxymethamphetamine was explored by U.S. Army Intelligence and later became popular as a recreational drug, which led to its scheduling as a controlled substance (Grob).
- Unlike conventional psychopharmacologic agents, psychedelics are administered only once or a few times in the context of psychotherapy and are meant to loosen defenses and facilitate insight (Grob).
- Set and setting, that is, the state of mind of a patient and the setting in which psychedelics are given, greatly influence the outcome of psychedelic treatment (Grob).
- Lengthy screening assessments and preparatory visits with trained facilitators enable patients to feel safe during treatment

---

sessions with psychedelics, and integrative sessions following treatment allow patients to make sense of their treatment experience (Osowski, Tipton).

NOTE: This list is the rapporteurs' summary of points made by the individual speakers identified, and the statements have not been endorsed or verified by the National Academies of Sciences, Engineering, and Medicine. They are not intended to reflect a consensus among workshop participants.

To understand the potential role of psychedelics in the future of psychiatry, understanding where the field has been and where it is now may be helpful, said Charles Grob, professor of psychiatry and pediatrics at the University of California, Los Angeles, School of Medicine.

The first archaeological evidence of shamanic use of mushrooms dates back to well over 7,000 years, said Grob. "We know from the anthropologic record that the use of plant hallucinogens was integral to the religious and medicinal practices and customs of the time," he said. However, the use of hallucinogenic plants for healing purposes was virtually unknown in the Western world until the early 1950s, when an amateur mycologist, R. Gordon Wasson, was invited by an Indigenous healer in central Mexico to participate in a healing ceremony. Wasson's account of his experience with "magic mushrooms" was published in *Life* magazine (Wasson, 1957), marking the first report of the mushrooms' psychedelic properties, said Grob.

Wasson sent the mushrooms to leading chemists around the world, including Albert Hoffman, who, only a decade or so earlier, had discovered that the synthetic chemical lysergic acid diethylamide (LSD) exerted powerful psychoactive effects. Hoffman, noted Grob, was also the first to identify psilocybin as the active alkaloid in the mushrooms. The British writer Aldous Huxley, best known as the author of the dystopian novel *Brave New World*, was also a proponent of psychedelic drugs during the 1950s, particularly in using them to "facilitate the passage of individuals from the end of life through dying," said Grob. Huxley corresponded about these mind-altering compounds with the British Canadian psychiatrist Humphrey Osmond, who coined the term "psychedelic," from the Greek word for mind manifesting. Other terms proposed included "hallucinogen," "entheogen" (accessing the divine within), "allucinari" (mind journeying, mind wandering, mind traveling), "psychotomimetic," "mysticomimetic," and "phantasticant." Even now, debate about nomenclature remains.

During the "golden era of psychedelic research" from the 1940s and 1960s, Grinspoon and Bakalar (1979) estimated that more than 1,000 published clinical papers detailed the experiences of some 40,000 patients treated with psychedelics, said Grob. Among the conditions targeted, some of the best outcomes were in the treatment of alcoholism, drug addiction, and PTSD, said Grob. Some studies have also indicated effectiveness in the treatment of chronic refractory obsessive-compulsive disorder (OCD), antisocial behavior, autism, depression, and profound reactive anxiety, such as the existential anxiety associated with terminal cancer, he said.

By the mid-to-late 1960s, however, psychedelics research unraveled as the drugs seeped out of research settings and began diffusing through the culture, said Grob. As they became increasingly linked to the politically active counterculture, Grob said they "became more and more outside the realm of what our society could deal with."

Unlike the plant-derived psychedelics, 3,4-Methylenedioxymethamphetamine (MDMA) was synthesized and patented by German chemists at Merck Pharmaceutical Company in 1912, but with the advent of hostilities in World War I, it was "put on a back shelf and forgotten," said Grob. Structurally similar to both mescaline and amphetamine, MDMA and related compounds captured the interest of U.S. Army Intelligence in the 1950s, but pursuit of these compounds came to an abrupt end when a participant in these investigations died. Clinical interest in MDMA resurfaced in the mid-1970s, but by the early 1980s it had become "wildly popular as a club drug," which led to its scheduling as a controlled substance, according to Grob. In the early 1990s, Grob and colleagues conducted the first Phase 1 study of MDMA to establish safety parameters (Grob et al., 1996).

THE PSYCHEDELIC PSYCHOPHARMACOLOGY PARADIGM

"Are we at the point where we might consider a paradigm shift [in psychopharmacology]?" asked Grob. Unlike conventional psychopharmacologic compounds, which are typically administered on a daily basis for weeks, months, or years, psychedelics are administered only once or a few times within the context of ongoing psychotherapy, he said. Conventional agents are also intended to ameliorate a pathological brain state and are not dependent on the patient's attitude or insight, while psychedelics loosen defenses, facilitate insight, and may induce a mystical experience. Most importantly, although conventional agents can be valuable for some people, many people's needs go unmet, said Grob.

Hallucinogens can be categorized as classic and non-classic, said Grob. Classic hallucinogens, such as mescaline, psilocin, and LSD have their primary effect on the serotonergic system and are primarily 5-HT_{2A} receptor agonists. Non-classic hallucinogens include MDMA, known more popularly as ecstasy or molly, ketamine, and ibogaine. MDMA is also known as an entactogen, which reflects its ability to promote affiliative social behavior (Nichols, 2022). Many of these compounds were originally discovered in plants and "have been used by Indigenous people since time immemorial," said Grob.

The subjective effects of psychedelics include stimulation of affect, enhanced capacity for insight and introspection, perceptual changes, and alterations of thought and time. It may feel like a waking, lucid dream, or a thematic vision that tells a story, said Grob. The psychedelic peak experience, a concept developed more than 50 years ago, includes a sense of awe and deeply felt reverence, a very positive mood, transcendence of time and space, and a sense of ineffability (Pahnke and Richards, 1966). According to Grob, "It's very difficult to put these experiences into words, endowing the user with a profound sense of meaning of their psychological and/or philosophical insight."

MDMA is relatively mild, easily controlled, and of moderate duration, said Grob, and has "the unique quality of facilitating profound empathy and compassion toward oneself and others." Combined with its ability to facilitate insight, introspection, and positive mood, he said MDMA has been "found to be very valuable within a psychotherapeutic context."

Looking to the future, Grob said optimizing safety and ethical parameters is critical. Two extrapharmacological variables—set and setting—greatly influence the outcome of treatment, he said. Set includes the personality, state of mind, vulnerabilities, expectations, and intentions of the person taking psychedelics. Setting refers to the physical, social, and cultural environment in which the compounds are taken. To ensure safe dosing, Grob said that the compounds should not be taken alone, but with a facilitator or therapist who can optimize the patient's safety. The potential for rapid commercialization presents additional challenges with respect to the safety of individuals who could benefit from these treatments. "We need to avoid the temptation to cut down on cost in order to maximize return on investment," which could put patients in jeopardy, he said. Grob also noted the need within the field to create opportunities for greater diversity among both investigators and study participants. These compounds offer great potential, he said, "but we need to avoid the mistakes of the past."

PERSONAL EXPERIENCES OF PSYCHEDELIC TREATMENT

A better understanding of the lived experiences of individuals treated with psychedelics is essential to ensure that future research efforts are designed to optimize the efficacy of these compounds in real-world settings. To ensure that the workshop reflected the patient perspective, two volunteers were asked to share their personal experiences of being treated with psychedelics—both the benefits of treatment and the challenges encountered in accessing this treatment. These narratives are meant to illustrate the types of responses individuals may have, but are not intended to represent the diversity of individuals who can benefit from this treatment nor the diversity of responses they may have.

Psilocybin for Major Depressive Disorder

Nora Osowski said she did not escape her family history of major depressive disorder, but as one of seven children in the family with two busy working parents, she got through her 20s and early 30s undiagnosed and without ever seeking treatment. By her mid-30s, after dealing with some health problems and the end of a long-term relationship, she sought treatment: first with tricyclic antidepressants, then selective serotonin reuptake inhibitors (SSRIs), norepinephrine reuptake inhibitors, and other atypical antidepressants. "I stuck with them for the prescribed amount of time"—at least 3 to 6 months for every class of antidepressant, she said, but "nothing worked."

Shortly before turning 39, she got married and immediately wanted to start a family, but 6 months into her pregnancy, she went into premature labor and lost her baby after an emergency cesarean section. On top of that loss, she went back to work at a stressful job. "Things just all came to a head and I experienced [such] a period of depression during which I couldn't get out of bed. I could no longer function," said Osowski.

A vacation to the Caribbean did not alleviate her depression, but on her way home from that trip, she decided to see if she could find something else to try in a clinical trial. Ketamine trials were no longer enrolling, but she found a psilocybin trial at Johns Hopkins University. "I would have tried anything at that time," Osowski said. "I was desperate."

Osowski went through the lengthy screening assessments, successfully enrolled, and began her preparatory visits with a social worker at Johns Hopkins who served as Osowski's session facilitator. During these visits, the social worker talked to her about her history and frame of mind and prepared her for what to expect in the trial. "She did an excellent job of making me feel safe and comfortable," including meeting with her in the treatment room, said Osowski.

Osowski described her first psilocybin session as "very intense." Encouraged to bring items from home, she brought her baby's blanket, ashes, photographs, and other meaningful belongings. Lying on the couch with eyeshades and headphones, listening to music (a playlist curated and standardized by the investigators and approved by an institutional review board), she said her mind was flooded with profound feelings of failure as a mother unable to protect her son. While it was a very emotional experience, she said, "I could look at that word 'failure' and feel very removed from it and objective." The two psilocybin treatment sessions were followed by integrative sessions, designed to enable Osowski to integrate insights realized during treatment. These sessions allowed her to process these memories further, which Osowski said was extremely valuable.

In her second session, she had an entirely different experience, highlighted by "a profound feeling of relaxation." She said that the entire experience of the trial brought her back in touch with her true core values and gave her the opportunity to reexamine her priorities and move beyond the negative thought patterns that had been so inescapable. She credited the trial with providing the spark she needed to go back to school and get a nursing degree. "I don't think that would have happened without my experience at Hopkins in the psilocybin trial," she said. "Psilocybin has had an enduring effect on the way I think, on how I've changed my priorities and my life," said Osowski.

MDMA-Assisted Psychotherapy for PTSD

Growing up in a household with a mentally unstable parent did little to prepare Lori Tipton, executive director of the Psychedelic Society of New Orleans, for the multiple traumas she would experience in her 20s. First, her brother died of a drug overdose. A few years later, in 2005, she discovered the bodies of her mother and two people her mother had murdered before committing suicide. The traumas kept on coming: only a month and a half later, Hurricane Katrina destroyed much of the Gulf Coast where Tipton lived, and the following year she was raped by someone she knew and trusted, became pregnant, and had an abortion.

Tipton said the next decade of her life was filled with the many symptoms of posttraumatic stress disorder (PTSD): anxiety and hypervigilance, mood swings, panic attacks, insomnia, suicidal ideation, and the inability to feel joy. She sought help from psychiatrists and other physicians, psychologists, social workers, therapists, physical therapists, an acupuncturist, a massage therapist, practitioners of deep-tissue bodywork known as Rolfing, and other alternative and homeopathic approaches to mental wellness. At times, she said, some of these modalities would temporarily relieve her symptoms, but "nothing really lasted, nothing addressed the core trauma."

In 2017, after reading about a study exploring the use of MDMA for the treatment of PTSD, Tipton applied and was accepted to participate in the Multidisciplinary Association for Psychedelic Studies (MAPS)[1] trial. The client-led therapy model being used in this study appealed to her because it gave her control over what would be discussed in the sessions. At several 1- to 2-hour preparatory sessions before her treatment, she talked with her two therapists about her goals. "I started thinking of them more as trauma

---

[1] To learn more about the MAPS Phase 3 MDMA-Assisted Therapy for PTSD study, see https://maps.org/mdma/ptsd/phase3 (accessed May 9, 2022).

doulas, who were there to create a safe environment for me to do the work of inner discovery and potential healing," she said. "It was clear to me that they weren't going to heal me, that I was going to have to do the work for myself, but that they were there to completely support my process." She added that these integrative sessions continued even after she had received the medication.

Tipton received MDMA three times over the course of approximately 3 months. She described these sessions as "very interesting and intense." "Taking a powerful empathogen and having two people there to completely support you is an incredibly healing event in itself," she said, adding that the effects of MDMA were also undeniable. "I felt embodied in a way that I hadn't in years because PTSD had robbed me of the ability to feel safe in my own body," she said.

A resurgence of memories flooded her mind during these sessions, said Tipton. "I felt everything—sadness, guilt, joy, loss, anger, surprise, understanding, confusion, and love. Everything and nothing." Recalling a vivid memory of playing with her brother when they were children allowed her to feel joy and elation, she said. "If that embodied experience of being with my brother was all I got out of the entire experience, it would have been completely worth it." She said she also recalled specifics about the murder scene at her mother's house that had been completely missing from her internal narrative of the event. "It wasn't like logically filling in the blank," but more like finding a section of a videotape that had been removed, she said.

As a result of these sessions, Tipton said she found a new perspective on life that had eluded her for years. "I felt as if I had been viewing the world through dirty lenses, and in those sessions the glass had been wiped clean." She learned to be more kind and patient with herself and others, to let go of the guilt she felt for people she had let down, and to cultivate love, understanding, and forgiveness for herself. Her personal therapist, whom she had continued to see throughout this time in the trial, commented that what Tipton had accomplished in less than 6 months would have taken decades to accomplish with traditional therapy. "I wouldn't say that MDMA-assisted therapy completely cured me of my PTSD, but when I completed the trial in 2018, I no longer qualified for the diagnosis and I still don't qualify for the diagnosis today," she said. "I don't suffer regularly from any of the symptoms that have plagued me for years."

3

Mechanisms of Action and Key Research Gaps for Psychedelics and Entactogens

HIGHLIGHTS

- While the therapeutic effects of classic psychedelics are not fully understood and likely multimodal, they are thought to reflect modulation of the serotonergic system, resulting in increased neuroplasticity and changes in connectivity (Gobbi).
- Psychedelics alter functional connectivity in the brain, which may explain their effects on consciousness, sensory processing, and the way people perceive themselves, the subjective experience, and the external world (Gobbi, Preller).
- A potential benefit of psychedelics is the possibility that they may cause long-term changes in sensory and associated networks with minimal drug exposure (Preller).
- "Psychoplastogens," including classic serotonergic psychedelics such as lysergic acid diethylamide and dimethyl tryptamine, emerges as a reference to a class of small-molecule drugs that may provide fast-acting and long-lasting antidepressant effects by inducing neuroplasticity through the growth of new dendrites and dendritic spines in the prefrontal cortex (Olson).
- It may be possible to make safer therapeutics by decoupling the hallucinogenic effects of psychoplastogenic compounds from their effects on neuroplasticity (Olson).
- The psychosocial context (also known as set and setting) of treatment delivery is an essential element of the efficacy

of psychedelic therapy, possibly by increasing psychological flexibility (Watts).

- Although substantial data support the idea that subjective effects of psychedelics are necessary to achieve full therapeutic benefits, more research is needed to answer this question definitively (Gonzalez-Maéso, Griffiths, Knudsen, Malenka, McClure-Begley, Watts).
- The synthesis of novel chemical compounds could help elucidate which targets engaged by psychedelics are essential to achieve therapeutic benefits (McClure-Begley).
- Observable traits, biomarkers of neuroplasticity, and genetic markers may be useful in predicting who will respond to psychedelic treatment (Griffiths, Knudsen, Krystal).
- Crafting a sophisticated and universal nomenclature for psychedelics could help advance the development of psychedelics for the treatment of psychiatric disorders (Knudsen, Malenka).

NOTE: This list is the rapporteurs' summary of points made by the individual speakers identified, and the statements have not been endorsed or verified by the National Academies of Sciences, Engineering, and Medicine. They are not intended to reflect a consensus among workshop participants.

Exploring the rich landscape of mechanisms that contribute to the therapeutic effects of psychedelics and entactogens will help guide the best use of these substances for different conditions, said Rita Valentino, director of the Division of Neuroscience and Behavior at the National Institute on Drug Abuse (NIDA). The fact that these effects cut across symptom domains suggests that the underlying neurobiological mechanisms probably extend beyond pharmacology to include complex interactions among environmental influences, social factors, and drug actions at the cellular, circuit, and network levels, said Valentino. In addition, their ability to have an enduring effect suggests that acute mechanisms may be very distinct from long-term mechanisms, she said.

Key questions that need to be answered include whether the hallucinogenic effects of psychedelics are essential for their therapeutic effects and whether plasticity, which has been linked to the mechanism of action of psychedelics, occurs at the level of cellular signaling, the synapse, circuit, or structure, said Valentino.

MOLECULAR MECHANISMS

Clinical studies have demonstrated that lysergic acid diethylamide (LSD) improves social behavior, increases empathy, and lessens anxiety and depression, said Gabriella Gobbi, a psychiatrist in the mood disorders program at the McGill University Health Centre and scientist at McGill University (Dolder et al., 2016; Gasser et al., 2015).While these effects are known to reflect modulation of the serotonergic system, Gobbi and colleagues have conducted preclinical research in rats and mice to try to understand at a molecular level LSD's mechanism of action, including the different receptors and parts of the brain that are affected.

Some of LSD's mechanisms of action are shared with selective serotonin reuptake inhibitor (SSRI) antidepressant medications such as Prozac, said Gobbi. For example, acute administration of both LSD and SSRIs decreases serotonin-firing activity by stimulating inhibitory autoreceptors (5-HT_{1A}), but repeated dosing results in desensitization of these receptors.

Gobbi has been particularly interested in how LSD enhances sociability in humans and the potential implications in autism and other neuro-psychiatric disorders. She and her colleagues have used multiple techniques in mouse models—electrophysiology, optogenetics, behavioral assessments, and molecular biology—to tease apart these effects. They showed that prosocial effects of LSD are mediated by increasing neurotransmission at two particular receptors—5-HT_{2A} and α-amino-3-hydroxy-5-methyl-4-isoxazole propionic acid (AMPA)—in the medial prefrontal cortex (mPFC), and that this process involves signaling through the mTOR complex in glutamatergic neurons (De Gregorio et al., 2021b). The mPFC is an area of the brain known to be important for social cognition, is implicated in autism spectrum disorder, and is rich with 5-HT_{2A} receptors, said Gobbi (Markopoulos et al., 2022).

She has also been exploring the mechanisms underlying LSD's ability to decrease anxiety (Gasser et al., 2015). Gobbi and colleagues have shown that in mice, chronic stress exposure causes a decrease in serotonin-firing activity and a loss of dendritic spines, which are restored with LSD treatment. Together these effects result in decreased stress-induced anxiety and increased neuroplasticity (De Gregorio et al., 2022).

One question that particularly intrigued Gobbi was why patients report such different experiences from LSD compared with SSRIs, given that they share similar mechanisms of action in the brain. Patients report that LSD and other psychedelics give new meaning to the experience of suffering, an alteration of consciousness, and a feeling of transcendence, said Gobbi. "We can't explain these effects only with the serotonin mechanism or the prefrontal cortex effect," she said. The psychedelics have properties not shared with the SSRIs.

"We can't study consciousness in mice or rats, but we can study these very important and intriguing nuclei in the brain called the reticular thalamic nuclei (RTN)," said Gobbi. The RTN is a thin sheet of gamma-aminobutyric acid (GABA)-ergic neurons that connects the thalamus to the cortex and is implicated in vigilance, sleep, and neuropsychiatric conditions, such as autism and schizophrenia, she said. More importantly, she said, brain imaging studies in humans have demonstrated that psychedelics alter this thalamocortical connection and may be linked to the experience of ego dissolution. Gobbi and colleagues demonstrated that LSD decreases firing of reticular thalamus neurons, which could explain alterations in consciousness (Inserra et al., 2021). A similar effect has been seen with psilocybin, she said (unpublished data). She added that because of the consciousness-altering effects of psychedelics, they should only be used in association with psychotherapy and in the presence of a trained therapist.

Circuit Mechanisms

When psychedelics stimulate various receptors in the brain, they change the activity of neurons, which results in changes in the way the brain processes information and interacts with the environment, said Katrin Preller, a research scientist at Yale University and the University of Zurich. Preller studies these processes at the circuit or network level, working from a model that focuses on the thalamus, a structure in the center of the brain that is responsible for filtering information. "This model suggests that under the influence of a psychedelic, the filtering function is reduced and, as a consequence, the cortex is overloaded with information, which then results in the symptoms that our participants are experiencing," she said (Preller et al., 2019).

Applying spectral dynamic causal modeling and global brain connectivity to resting-state functional magnetic resonance imaging (fMRI) data, she and her colleagues have shown that LSD and psilocybin change connectivity patterns in the brain, resulting in disintegration of activity in what are normally highly integrated brain regions. More specifically, they observed increased sensory processing in combination with decreased processing capacity in brain areas responsible for making sense of that information and relating it to memories.

"This counterbalance of increased sensory processing and decreased association processing may explain why participants under the influence of psychedelics have visual alterations, but also why they may be able to perceive themselves and the world in a different way, because they are integrating information differently than they usually do," said Preller. She and Franz Vollenweider of the University of Zurich have hypothesized that psychedelics may be beneficial for people with depression or substance use disorders because they are able to experience themselves and the world in a different way, which allows them to move past rigid thinking patterns and negative self-impressions (Vollenweider and Preller, 2020). More trials in depression and alcohol use disorder are planned to test this hypothesis, she said.

Preller added that while there are fewer data available on the circuit-level changes under 3,4-Methylenedioxymethamphetamine (MDMA), some studies suggest that in comparison with LSD and psilocybin, MDMA causes similar disintegration of associated brain regions as well as no disintegration of sensory brain networks.

As mentioned earlier, one of the potential benefits of psychedelics for the treatment of psychiatric disorders is the hope that they will introduce long-term changes after minimal drug exposure. However, Preller said that little is known about long-term changes at the network level. One study demonstrated differentiation between sensory and association networks a month after administration of a single dose of psilocybin (Barrett et al., 2020), but another study failed to show significant network changes at 3 months (McCulloch et al., 2022).

Many knowledge gaps remain in understanding the effects of psyche-delics at the circuit level and optimizing their use as therapies, said Preller. These include (1) whether circuit-level changes contribute to clinical efficacy; (2) whether there are transdiagnostic circuit-level changes, for example, whether the same changes contribute to clinical efficacy in depression and alcohol use disorder; (3) how much interindividual variability exists; (4) what the optimal dose is for these substances; and (5) how specific the network effects are across different substances.

Psychoplastogenic Effects

Stress-related neuropsychiatric disorders, such as depression, PTSD, and substance use disorder, can be resistant to treatment with currently available drugs that aim to rectify chemical imbalances in the brain, said David Olson, associate professor of chemistry, biochemistry and molecular medicine at the University of California, Davis. Olson and colleagues have pioneered a new approach, which uses small-molecule drugs to selectively modulate neural circuits. This approach targets atrophy of neurons in the prefrontal cortex (PFC)—a hallmark of these illnesses—by changing the structure of the cortical neurons that tend to atrophy in response to chronic stress, said Olson.

Olson calls these molecules psychoplastogens because they induce structural neuroplasticity through the growth of new dendrites and dendritic spines, which are the sites of excitatory synapses in the brain. Unlike the more traditional antidepressants, such as SSRIs, which take weeks or months to show efficacy and are ineffective for about a third of patients, psychoplastogens should produce long-lasting effects after a single administration, said Olson.

Classic serotonergic psychedelics, such as LSD and dimethyl tryptamine (DMT), were among the first psychoplastogens Olson and his team studied. As shown in Figure 3-1, both of these compounds promote the growth of neuronal dendritic spines and increased complexity of dendritic arbors in comparison with neurons treated with a vehicle control (VEH) (Ly et al., 2018). These effects were eliminated by blocking the serotonin 2A receptor or downstream kinases, including tyrosine protein kinase B (TrkB) and mTOR.

In vivo studies showed similar results, said Olson. In rats, a single injection of DMT produced a profound increase in dendritic spine density

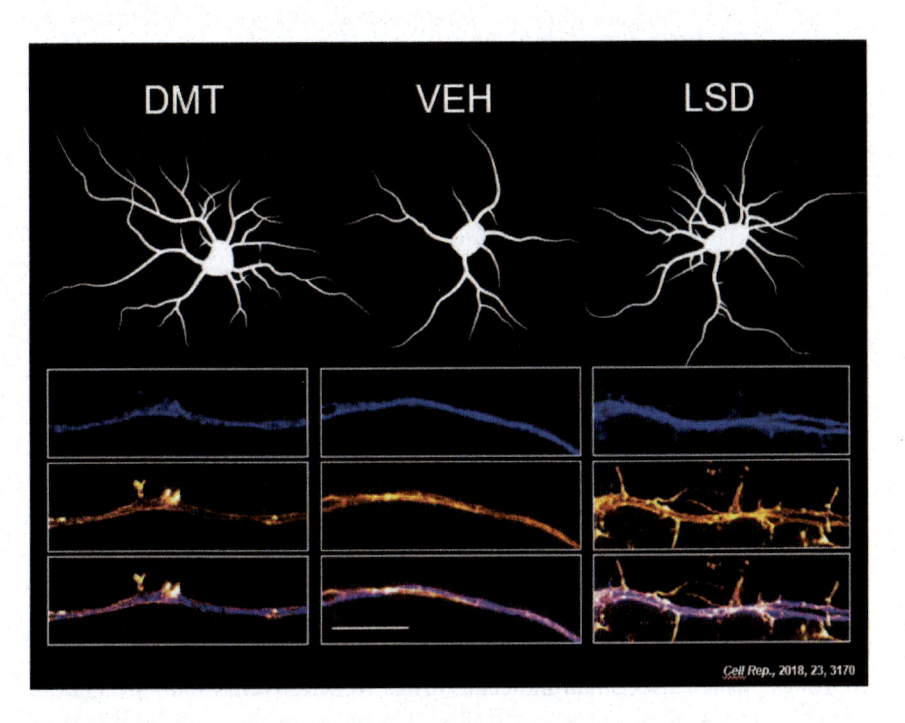

FIGURE 3-1 Psychedelics promote dendritic spine growth in vitro. Representative tracings (top) and high-resolution microscopy (bottom) of cortical neurons treated with LSD or DMT show substantially more complex dendritic arbors and increased growth of dendritic spines and filopodia-like structures in comparison with neurons treated with VEH.

NOTES: DMT = N,N-dimethyl tryptamine; LSD = lysergic acid diethylamide; VEH = vehicle control.

SOURCES: Presented by David Olson, March 29, 2022; data from Ly et al., 2018.

in the PFC as well as long-lasting functional changes in these neurons. He added that these studies have been replicated and extended by several groups, including one study where a single dose of psilocybin was shown to cause increased spine density that lasted for at least a month (Shao et al., 2021). Using $5\text{-}HT_{2A}$ receptor knockout animals, Olson and colleagues have shown that this functional and structural plasticity is mediated by $5\text{-}HT_{2A}$ receptors.

One of the promising aspects of psychoplastogens is their ability to work across indications, which Olson said reflects the fact that they target the PFC, a critical hub in the brain. PFC circuitry modulates drug-seeking behavior, motivation, mood, the expression of fear, and many other aspects of brain function that underlie depression and related disorders, he said. In animal studies, Olson's lab has demonstrated profound antidepressant effects of psychoplastogens, which are completely blocked by the $5\text{-}HT_{2A}$ receptor antagonist ketanserin. Another active area of research in Olson's lab is the potential use of psychoplastogens to restore atrophied neurons in neurodegenerative conditions, such as Alzheimer's disease. He added that $5\text{-}HT_{2A}$ receptors are expressed not only on cortical neurons but also on the immune cells in the brain, microglia, and astrocytes, raising the possibility that psychedelics may have anti-inflammatory effects on the brain.

"These studies suggest that the $5\text{-}HT_{2A}$ receptor plays a critical role in both the psychoplastogenic effects and the beneficial behavioral effects of psychedelics in preclinical models," said Olson. However, the $5\text{-}HT_{2A}$ receptor is also known to mediate the hallucinogenic effects of these drugs, he said. To create a safer therapeutic for a larger patient population, he wanted to know if it was possible to decouple the hallucinogenic effects of psychedelics from their effects on structural and functional neuroplasticity and their beneficial behavioral effects. His group has been working with a compound called 6-methoxy-DMT, which is not hallucinogenic, unlike the closely related and highly hallucinogenic compound 5-methoxy-DMT. "What was really exciting to us is that 6-methoxy-DMT is still a potent psychoplastogen, can produce the growth of new neurites, and can promote increased spine density," said Olson, adding that these effects seem to be mediated by the $5\text{-}HT_{2A}$ receptor.

Olson and colleagues have now engineered a novel compound called tabernanthalog (TBG), a non-toxic analog of ibogaine and 5-methoxy-DMT (Cameron et al., 2021). They showed in mice that TBG has a low hallucinogenic profile but provides a profound increase in spine formation and beneficial effects on neuronal structure and function. They also showed that these effects were blocked in $5\text{-}HT_{2A}$ knockout neurons. "This suggests some type of functional selectivity," said Olson. "We can engage the $5\text{-}HT_{2A}$ receptor and turn on plasticity or hallucinogenic effects, but we don't have to turn on both at the same time."

TBG was also shown to have antidepressant effects in wild type but not 5-HT_{2A} knockout mice, and these therapeutic effects require spinogenesis, which suggests a causal relationship between structural plasticity in the PFC and sustained antidepressant effects, said Olson.

Several unanswered questions remain, including the duration of the therapeutic effects and whether polypharmacology plays a role and could be used to tailor treatment for different indications, said Olson. Finally, he noted the importance of developing translatable biomarkers of the structural changes in the brain that are induced by psychoplastogens.

PSYCHOSOCIAL CONTEXTS AS ESSENTIAL TREATMENT ELEMENTS

As highlighted earlier in Chapter 2 by individuals who have undergone psychedelic treatment, the preparation and integration sessions with therapists are key to a positive therapeutic outcome. Indeed, said clinical psychologist Rosalind Watts, psychosocial contexts (also referred to as set and setting) are essential treatment elements. "You can't separate the drug from the context," said Watts, who was the clinical lead for the psilocybin trial at Imperial College London and is the clinical director of the Synthesis Institute.[1] "One of the biggest problems in psychedelic therapy at the moment is a widespread overestimating of the importance of the drug and an underestimation of the non-drug elements," she said.

Watts said that without these elements, psychedelic therapy may be ineffective or even dangerous. Psychedelics do not work like other drugs, she said. "The participant is not a passive recipient and the degree of trust they feel toward themselves, the therapist, and the substance will determine whether the drug works at all and how safe it is." Lacking this trust, she said, patients may be "unable to surrender to the experience and make the most of it."

Watts acknowledged that there is little research teasing out the benefits and mechanisms of these non-drug elements, in part because it would be unethical to provide psychedelics without them. Brain imaging combined with qualitative research has indicated, however, that an overarching mechanism that contributes to treatment efficacy is psychological flexibility, said Watts.

Watts has proposed a simplified model informed by six psychological flexibility concepts as well as a thematic analysis of the qualitative experiences of participants in psychedelic therapy trials (see Figure 3-2). She calls this model "Accept, Connect, Embody," or ACE (Watts and Luoma, 2020).

---

[1] To learn more about the Synthesis Institute, see https://www.synthesisinstitute.com (accessed May 14, 2022).

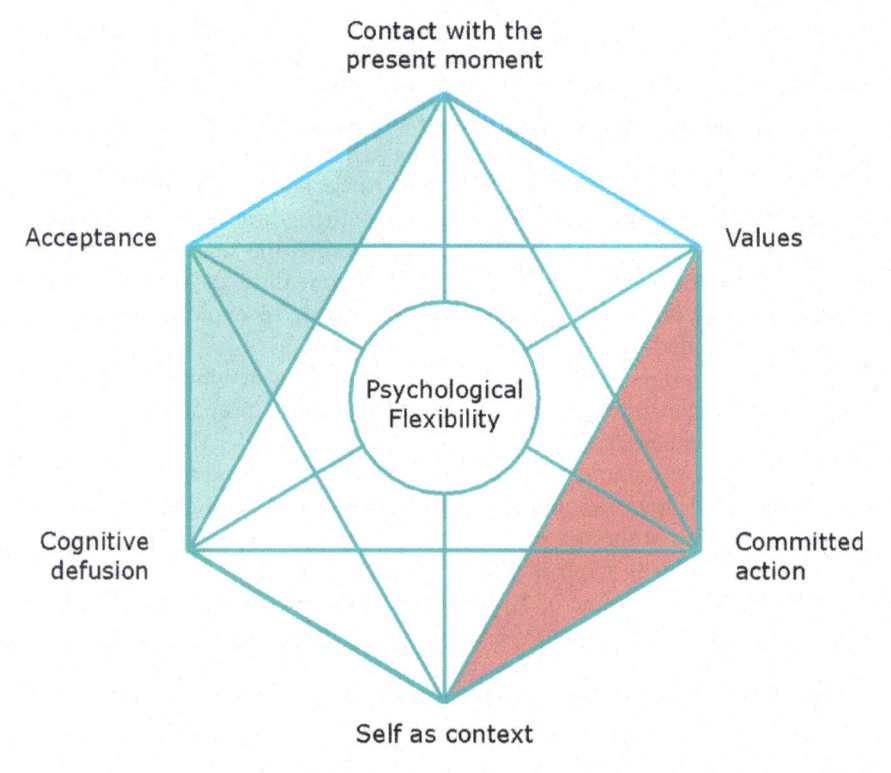

FIGURE 3-2 Psychological flexibility combines six core processes of Acceptance Commitment Therapy (ACT): connecting with the present moment, accepting and being willing to feel emotions, connecting with one's values, committing oneself to values-based behaviors and actions, defusing negative thoughts, and observing oneself beyond simply one's thoughts and feelings.
NOTE: To learn more about the six core process of ACT, see https://contextualscience.org/the_six_core_processes_of_act (accessed May 14, 2022).
SOURCES: Presented by Rosalind Watts, March 29, 2022; Hayes, 1999.

From being a guide in so many psilocybin therapy sessions, Watts said she has come to believe that these three elements determine the effectiveness of psilocybin treatment for depression.

She simplified the model into its three main elements: acceptance, connection, and embodiment. "Acceptance is the most important aspect for avoiding a bad trip" said Watts, "it is all about being able to let go and feel whatever comes up in the session." The preparation and integration sessions reassure patients that even uncomfortable or frightening experiences during the treatment sessions provide the potential for learning and change and that they will be safe. Connectedness focuses on an individual's ability to stay with the emotional content of what they are experiencing. Connecting these experiences to new insights at the time of treatment and in integrative sessions after the treatment sessions helps patients derive meaning from the experience. "The most common insight from people is they realize everything is interconnected, rather than being separate," said Watts. Embodiment refers to the experience as it is felt in the body, said Watts. "Often people experience some kind of insight into their difficulties through for example a tight feeling in their chest. . . . There is the sense that we hold our traumas in our bodies, and people are able to really access those pockets of held trauma that have crystalized and are able to explore and release [them]," she added.

The preparation sessions are about building trust, which takes time, said Watts. Visualization exercises are often used to prepare patients for the psilocybin experience. For example, Watts might offer the analogy of a pearl dive. "They imagine they're swimming out to sea, and they dive under the surface and down to the bottom of the sea and look around. It's all about going toward the spikey oyster shells at the bottom of the sea rather than swimming away from them; opening the oysters up and looking for pearls, and then swimming up to the surface with this new outlook on life."

Embodiment also requires extensive preparation, said Watts, adding that having two guides is important and that the sessions should be videotaped. Setting boundaries with regard to touch should be done in advance. Music is another critical part of the psilocybin experience and can be thought of as the "third therapist," she said. "It's really important to have a good playlist." It can help people be in their bodies and can open them up to emotions that might otherwise be resisted.

The integration sessions are about finding meaning in the experience, said Watts. Some patients have clear insights, but for others, very careful and sensitive non-directed therapeutic support can help patients make a narrative of what they learned through the experience, which helps them to continue benefiting from the treatment even after the "afterglow" ends, she said.

Watts described a psilocybin trial at the Imperial College London, which was a randomized trial comparing two groups that both had two guides and music mediation, preparation, and integration sessions. One group received 25 milligrams of psilocybin while the other group received 1 milligram of psilocybin (as placebo) plus a course of the SSRI antidepressant escitalopram (Carhart-Harris et al., 2021). No significant differences were found between the two groups on the primary outcome measure, measuring symptoms of depression. However, as the leader of the clinical team, Watts spoke with all participants. Among those in the antidepressant group, many told her that the antidepressants were not responsible for the benefits they experienced. "What they described as profound was the experience of having two therapists, two days of sitting with music, and having space for the emergence of what is referred to in psychedelic therapy as the inner healer that we all have within us," said Watts. "So I would say that we mustn't underestimate the importance of the care and the connectedness that psychedelic therapy offers people, and how much of an impact that has on the outcomes."

Beyond this trial, Watts cited several research studies that have demonstrated the importance of context (Carhart-Harris et al., 2018), emotional breakthrough (Roseman et al., 2019), and the quality of the acute psychedelic experience (Roseman et al., 2018) in achieving therapeutic efficacy, as well as the potential benefits of providing psychedelics in group settings, known as psychedelic communitas (Kettner et al., 2021). While there has been little research to prove that the drug and the psychosocial context are inseparable, she highlighted the fact that many people take psychedelics recreationally but describe no therapeutic benefits. Watts said she views psychedelics as compounds that can amplify psychedelic-assisted therapy, but that without the psychological flexibility framework, the benefits are lost very quickly.

LINKING BIOLOGICAL, PSYCHOLOGICAL, AND CLINICAL EFFECTS OF PSYCHEDELICS: RESEARCH GAPS AND OPPORTUNITIES

Although evidence has been accumulating to support the therapeutic use of psychedelics and entactogens, critical research gaps remain, said John Krystal, chair of the department of psychiatry at Yale University. To further develop these agents for the treatment of psychiatric disorders, Krystal said further research is needed in three critical areas: (1) translating molecular and circuit effects of psychedelics into clinical benefits; (2) identifying the critical psychological and psychosocial treatment elements that underlie clinical benefits; and (3) understanding the therapeutic importance of psychedelic effects.

The serotonin 2A receptor is known to be the main molecular target of classic psychedelics, but Robert Malenka, Pritzker Professor of Psychiatry and Behavioral Sciences at Stanford University, suggested that while necessary, it may not be sufficient. "It may be much more complicated than activating serotonin 2A receptors to get therapeutic benefits," he said Another still open question is whether post-acute effects of psychedelics are mediated by this receptor, said Javier González-Maeso, professor of physiology and biophysics at the Virginia Commonwealth University School of Medicine. If the mechanisms of the acute and postacute effects are different, it may be possible to achieve therapeutic effects without hallucinations, he said.

Is the Subjective Experience Necessary?

Related to this question and also unanswered is whether the psychedelic effects are necessary to achieve therapeutic effects, said González-Maeso. Roland Griffiths, professor of psychiatry and neurosciences at the Johns Hopkins University School of Medicine, asserted that the subjective effects reflect the underlying neurobiology and are necessary for full and enduring therapeutic effects. Historical, anecdotal, and qualitative data support this view, he said. As was pointed out by Watts and described by Nora Osowski and Lori Tipton in Chapter 2, clinical studies have shown that participants attach deep meaning and significance to their psychedelic experiences, including a sense of connectedness and unity, said Griffiths. He suggested that something about these experiences is integral to meaning making[2] and the construction of a changed narrative. In addition, he said it has been shown experimentally that features of the mystical-type experience are predictive of enduring positive changes going forward.

Malenka said while he also believes the subjective experience is critically important for therapeutic benefits, much of the evidence is correlative. Griffiths suggested one approach that would disprove the importance of subjective effects experimentally: administration of psychedelics to individuals rendered fully unconscious. If participants in such a study had no memory of the psychedelic experience yet had full and lasting therapeutic efficacy, subjective effects would seem irrelevant. Although such an experiment could be difficult, Malenka said, "If there is an experiment to be done that disproves your hypothesis, you should do it. In fact, you are morally bound to do it."

Malenka suggested that another experiment that could help tease out the importance of hallucinogenic or mystical experiences would be to compare treatment of depression using lisuride, the non-hallucinogenic analog of LSD, versus psilocybin or LSD in combination with adjunctive psychotherapy. An even more difficult experiment would be to block the subjective experience by administering the 5-HT_{2A} antagonist ketanserin before psilocybin or LSD. If under that pharmacologic condition LSD or psilocybin still showed a therapeutic benefit, "that would be a very powerful result that would actually change the game enormously," said Malenka.

Whether the therapeutic benefits result from the drug's interaction at the receptor or from the whole therapeutic session is a "strange dichotomy," said Gitte Moos Knudsen, professor of neurology and chair of the Neurobiology Research unit at the University of Copenhagen and Rigshospitalet, Denmark. "What we experience makes us who we are and we are our

---

[2] Meaning making is the "process by which people interpret situations, events, objects, or discourses, in the light of their previous knowledge and experience" (Zittoun and Brinkmann, 2012).

brains," she said. She noted that there are large individual differences in how people react to these substances and suggested that there may be an epigenetic explanation that ties together an individual's experience with the pharmacological effects at the 5-HT$_{2A}$ receptor site.

Particularly intriguing, she said, is the observation that many people who have mystical experiences with their first exposure to psychedelics have a similar experience on a second occasion months later, whereas those who do not have a mystical experience the first time usually do not have one the second time either. Griffiths agreed that there appear to be real individual differences but said there are also considerable within-subject differences.

Griffiths added that people who are less open to the psychedelic experience seem to struggle more with it, which results in a strong selection bias with respect to the people who decide to participate in these studies. Krystal said he saw similar struggles among participants in ketamine trials, which may be related to temperament. "People who were very frightened by losing control were more likely to be frightened and have a difficult experience during ketamine [treatment] than people who found the ketamine experience interesting, engaging, or even exciting," he said. Knudsen pointed to the known relationship between personality and cerebral 5-HT$_{2A}$ receptor density, noting that studies have shown a correlation between the receptor density and both neuroticism and openness. Knudsen suggested that there may be observable traits that could be used to predict who would benefit from the treatment.

Understanding the Linkage Between Mechanism and Effect

A disconnect exists between basic science and clinical work, in part because there are no good animal models for neuropsychiatric disease, said Olson. "These are uniquely human conditions," he said. Animal studies can, however, be used to look at specific behavioral readouts of certain circuitry activation and to assess the effects of environmental changes, he said.

Krystal added that "there is a tendency to think about the effects of these drugs as either working through their molecular or synaptic plasticity or through cognitive mechanisms." But there may also be both component benefits and component risks associated with each of these mechanisms, and these effects may be additive, he said. Griffiths noted that serious toxicities are associated with psychedelics. Yet, he nonetheless questioned the ethics of withholding the possibility of a life-changing experience from someone who would otherwise not have such an experience.

Also with regard to plasticity, Malenka said that differentiating drug-induced from psychotherapy-induced plasticity is a false dichotomy. "I believe that certain forms of psychotherapy are powerful therapeutic agents of change that work by modifying spines, synapses, and circuits in the brain, just in very complex ways that are much harder to understand than giving a single drug that has one or multiple molecular targets that we can manipulate," he said.

Tristan McClure-Begley, program manager at the Defense Advanced Research Projects Agency (DARPA), proposed diversifying the chemical space around psychedelics as an alternative approach toward understanding the mechanisms underlying their therapeutic effects. "We've been tossing around concepts that can really be broken down into two separate questions," he said. One is whether subjective effects are necessary for therapeutic effects of psychedelics; the other is whether the targets engaged by psychedelics represent "therapeutic gateways in their own right that may share some, but not all, of the mechanistic aspects of classic psychedelics for therapeutic use."

To answer this second question will require the synthesis of novel chemical compounds, said McClure-Begley. Most known chemotypes engage neurotransmitter receptors in an unbiased fashion and are indiscriminate with respect to the downstream signaling pathways they activate, he said. By contrast, he proposed designing and testing novel chemical matter with predictable and reliable pharmacokinetics that selectively engage downstream signaling with minimal off-target effects. For example, a drug that engages 5-HT_{2A} but does not cause the psychedelic experience might not be useful taken a few times in guided therapy sessions. However, it could be useful as a more traditional psychopharmacologic agent, said McClure-Begley.

He noted that there are known non-psychedelic analogues of some hallucinogens, such as LSD. Adding to our toolbox in terms of molecular diversity could allow us to see, for example, to what degree signaling bias is necessary or sufficient to engage mechanisms that cause certain behavioral effects, he said. "We could also, at the same time, be talking about a completely different therapeutic mechanism of action compared to what is possible with classic psychedelics," said McClure-Begley.

Griffiths added that "our understanding of the differences among these different existing psychedelic compounds is embarrassingly primitive." A few preclinical studies have provided clues, said Krystal. For example, the spines produced during psilocybin treatment last longer than those created during ketamine infusions, he said, although the mechanisms underlying these differences are unclear. González-Maeso added that studies with 1-(2,5-dimethoxy-4-iodophenyl)-2-aminopropane (DOI), a psychedelic structurally similar to but more potent than mescaline affects gene expression and chromatic organization after a single dose, which does not happen with ketamine. He suggested that the longer duration of effects from psilocybin and other classic psychedelics may be related to gene expression and plasticity.

While psychedelics are known to induce changes in brain connectivity, how long these changes last remains an important unanswered question, said Preller. She suggested that studies comparing the effects of classic psychedelics with ketamine could be valuable to increase understanding of trans-drug mechanisms. Olson mentioned that all of these drugs produce similar effects on corticostructural plasticity, but they have distinct targets, and their effects persist for different periods of time. "What that really suggests is that they can engage a similar biochemical pathway," he said. For example, TrkB and mTOR activation seems to be critical for all of these agents, which suggests new therapeutic targets distinct from 5-HT_{2A} receptor activation, he said.

Another important question to be answered is where in the brain these drugs are active, said Malenka. "I don't believe the whole story is the PFC, and in the PFC it's going to depend on which class of neurons are being modified and what they are connected to," he said. Moreover, the signaling bias you want in a therapeutic agent will not be uniform throughout the brain," said Malenka. Figuring out which circuits are being modified in which brain areas could help bridge the gap between preclinical and clinical research using human brain imaging and resting state functional connectivity studies, he said.

Valentino added that some LSD users report flashbacks of hallucinogenic experiences many years later. The molecular mechanisms underlying these flashbacks are unclear, said Gobbi, but may involve the thalamus, as well as the hippocampus and entorhinal cortex, which are important for autobiographical memory.

Predicting Responsiveness to Psychedelic Treatment

Knudsen pointed to the emerging evidence from animal studies that psychedelics induce neuroplasticity that may be associated with the beneficial treatment effects. To investigate this further in humans, possible markers of neuroplasticity could include levels of serum brain derived neurotrophic factor (BDNF), hippocampal volume assessed with magnetic resonance imaging (MRI), assessment of glutamate levels using mass spectroscopy, molecular neuroimaging of the synaptic vesicle protein 2A (SV2A) using positron emission tomography (PET), or electroencephalogram-based visual potentials, she said. She also urged the development of other novel PET tracers to identify the optimal molecular target.

With respect to SV2A imaging, Krystal cited a recent pilot study that, in a secondary analysis, showed that in depressed patients with reduced synaptic density, but not in those with normal synaptic density, a single dose of ketamine increased SV2A binding, and these increases were correlated with reduced depression severity (Holmes et al., 2022). While ketamine produced dissociative symptoms in patients with and without evidence of synaptic deficits, dissociative symptoms correlated with clinical improvement and synaptic increases only in those patients who had initial synaptic deficits. While ketamine is not a psychedelic drug, these results suggest that dissociative symptoms do not mediate clinical benefits, but rather serve as a marker of changes in circuit function that are permissive of adaptive plasticity in subgroups of patients, said Krystal.

Griffiths also suggested investigating genetic markers for sensitivity to transcendent experiences, noting that data to address this question are currently insufficient.

Studies by Alex Kwan and colleagues at Yale have demonstrated profound sex differences in the increase in spine density following a single dose of psilocybin, and similar sex differences have been seen in preclinical studies of ketamine and other psychedelics, said Olson (Shao et al., 2021). In small human studies, however, Preller and colleagues have not observed sex differences in the response to psychedelics.

Standardizing Nomenclature

As was alluded to in Chapter 1, questions remain about nomenclature, said Malenka. He said that addressing this issue and developing a more sophisticated language among researchers, government agencies, and philanthropic organizations will grow in importance as the field develops. The term "psychedelic" itself is problematic when used to encompass the different classes of compounds that were discussed at this workshop, said Malenka. For example, he argued that classic serotonin 2A hallucinogenic ligands, such as LSD and psilocybin, are mechanistically and subjectively quite different from entactogens such as MDMA. In addition, the dissociative anesthetic ketamine, which is often lumped together with classic hallucinogens, most likely works through different mechanisms, he said.

Malenka said more rigorous and sophisticated language is also needed when discussing concepts such as plasticity. There are maladaptive forms of plasticity that involve spine changes and changes in the dendritic tree and in circuit dynamics, as well as decades of research showing that drugs of abuse can cause structural changes in different parts of the brain. Knudsen agreed on the need for more rigorous nomenclature when it comes to definitions of the term "psychedelics" and suggested the neuroscience-based nomenclature introduced by the European College of Neuropsychopharmacology.[3]

---

[3] To learn more about the neuroscience-based nomenclature published by the European College of Neuropsychopharmacology, see https://www.ecnp.eu/research-innovation/nomenclature (accessed May 25, 2022).

4

Advancing Clinical Development: Challenges and Opportunities

HIGHLIGHTS

- While psychotherapy is essential to the efficacy and safety of psychedelic treatment, it has not been rigorously defined or standardized for this use (Muñiz).
- The Food and Drug Administration does not regulate the practice of medicine, including off-label prescribing of medications or psychotherapy, but it may require a risk evaluation and mitigation strategy or include recommendations in the labeling of a drug (Muñiz).
- Assessing the efficacy of psychedelics may be confounded by expectancy bias, functional unblinding, and the tendency of these drugs to heighten participant suggestibility (Muñiz).
- Psychological support used in psychedelic therapy trials—using two therapists and including video recordings—is designed to facilitate treatment and ensure safety, yet specifics of how these elements should be incorporated have not been defined (de Boer, Levine, Muñiz).
- Set and setting are important elements of psychedelic therapy, although required parameters have been inadequately studied and defined (Muñiz, Rao).
- To minimize bias despite the difficulty of blinding a study of psychedelic therapy, researchers have explored several strategies, including using active controls, subperceptual doses as

controls, blinding questionnaires, and blinding of raters, yet each approach has challenges (Colloca, Muñiz).

- Research strategies that examine the necessity of the conscious experience for achieving therapeutic benefits include using non-psychedelic psychoplastogens or sedating patients before treatment (Raison).
- If the conscious experience proves to be an essential element of treatment, more research will be needed to determine the optimal parameters for achieving it (Raison).
- Clinical trials of methylenedioxymethamphetamine-assisted therapy for posttraumatic stress disorder indicate strong efficacy with a large treatment effect (Reiff).
- Clinical trials of psilocybin for treatment-resistant depression suggest robust and durable responses in many, but not all, participants (de Boer, Levine, Reiff).
- Increasing diversity among participants and therapists in clinical trials of psychedelics is important to ensure access to these modalities across diverse communities (de Boer).
- Psilocybin produced significant reductions in depression and anxiety symptoms among patients with life-threatening illnesses and in the treatment of substance use disorders (Reiff).

NOTE: This list is the rapporteurs' summary of points made by the individual speakers identified, and the statements have not been endorsed or verified by the National Academies of Sciences, Engineering, and Medicine. They are not intended to reflect a consensus among workshop participants.

The novelty of psychedelics and entactogens for treating psychiatric disorders paired with marked psychoactive effects of these drugs presents unique challenges to evaluations of efficacy and will require modifications to standard clinical trial design, said Gerard Sanacora, Gross Professor of Psychiatry at the Yale University School of Medicine, Director of the Yale Depression Research Program, and Co-Director of the Interventional Psychiatry Program at Yale-New Haven Hospital. Indeed, the high degree of enthusiasm and anticipation for psychedelics is "beyond anything we have ever seen with any unapproved psychiatric drug," said Javier Muñiz, Commander in the U.S. Public Health Service and associate director for Therapeutic Review in the Division of Psychiatry, Office of New Drugs at the Food and Drug Administration (FDA).

Muñiz noted that although hundreds of papers were published between the 1960s and 1990s on the use of psychedelics, most had methodologic problems that would not meet today's rigorous regulatory standards. In the past 20, however, he said there has been a resurgence in high-quality research, as illustrated in Figure 4-1. Within FDA, Investigational New Drug Applications (NDAs) have also surged in the past few years, said Muñiz. However, he noted that in an evidence-based summary of literature on the clinical application of psychedelic drugs in psychiatric disorders, Reiff and colleagues concluded that while randomized controlled trials support the efficacy of 3,4-Methylenedioxymethamphetamine (MDMA) for the treatment of posttraumatic stress disorder (PTSD) and psilocybin for the treatment of depression and cancer-related anxiety, the data are currently insufficient for FDA approval of these drugs for routine clinical use (Reiff et al., 2020).

When FDA reviews an NDA, they look for evidence of both safety and efficacy, said Muñiz. Features of FDA's existing regulatory framework that are most relevant to psychedelic drugs include the requirement that a study permits a valid comparison, that bias on the part of both participants and observers is minimized, and that the methods of assessment are well defined and reliable, he said.

CONFOUNDERS TO EFFICACY ASSESSMENTS

Muñiz mentioned several factors associated with psychedelics that confound efficacy assessment. For example, psychedelic treatment is provided by highly engaged therapists and monitors, which in and of itself may be therapeutic, as mentioned earlier. In addition, Muñiz noted that both patients and therapists often have elevated expectations about efficacy, fueled in part by highly favorable media coverage; elaborate intervention protocols may further increase the placebo response. There are also issues related to blinding because the dramatic responses some people experi-

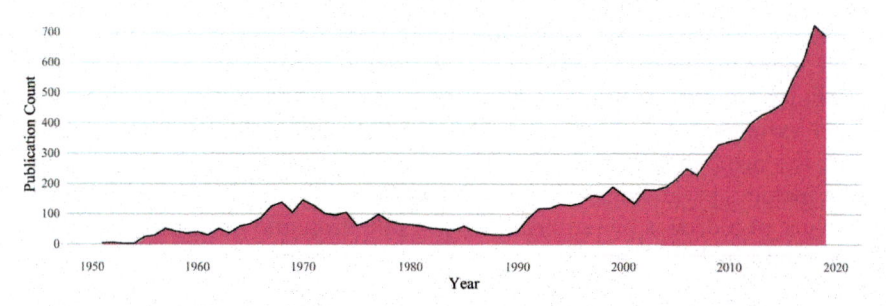

FIGURE 4-1 Psychedelic scientific publications by year. The number of psychedelic publications has increased substantially in the past 20 years, according to the web of science publication count.
SOURCES: Presented by Javier Muñiz, March 30, 2022; Petranker et al., 2020.

ence when taking psychedelics may result in what is known as functional unblinding, said Muñiz. Finally, he noted that psychedelics appear to have unique suggestibility properties, which can complicate the reliability of participant reporting.

Muñiz highlighted three challenges that merit further consideration from a regulatory perspective: (1) the inclusion of psychotherapy as a treatment element, (2) the importance of set and setting, and (3) the challenge of making valid comparisons and minimizing biases.

Psychotherapy as a Treatment Element

Psychotherapy is integral to maximizing the treatment effect and ensuring safety, said Muñiz, but it has not been rigorously defined and standardized for use during psychedelic treatment. It is typically involved at three stages of psychedelic trials—at the preparatory stage to help build rapport and establish goals and intentions; during the in-drug treatment sessions to facilitate the sessions and reduce adverse psychological reactions; and in the weeks and months following the administration of psychedelics to process and integrate the experience and ensure psychological stability. "However, we don't know which features of the psychotherapy intervention are critical for efficacy or what minimum components of the psychotherapeutic intervention are necessary to ensure safety," said Muñiz, adding that this information is critical for labeling. For example, Sanacora mentioned that if psychedelics are inducing long-term plasticity in humans similar to what the preclinical studies show, it might be better to implement psychotherapeutic augmentation strategies after giving participants a chance to recover from the treatment.

To fully tease out the safety and efficacy contributions of psychotherapy would require well-done factorial studies, said Muñiz. He noted, however, that while FDA regulates labeling, it does not regulate the practice of medicine, which includes off-label prescribing and psychotherapy. They have, however, written labels specifying that a drug should be used only in conjunction with another mode of therapy, said Muñiz. For example, the label for naltrexone as a treatment for alcohol and opioid dependence states that the drug should be part of a "comprehensive management program that includes psychological support." Another approach FDA uses to ensure safe use of a drug is by requiring a risk evaluation and mitigation strategy[1] that could include elements such as provider training or certification, said Muñiz, noting that this requirement must not be unduly burdensome to patients or the health care system. He added that while risk evaluation and mitigation strategy (REMS) is usually proposed by a sponsor, FDA is con-

---

[1] 21 U.S. Code Section 355-1.

sidering developing a REMS program for psychedelics given the complexity of the risks associated with these agents.

Steven Levine, senior vice president of patient access and medical affairs at COMPASS Pathways, noted that the model of psychological support used in psychedelic therapy was designed not to provide psychotherapy per se, but to accompany, facilitate, and ensure safety within trials. Video recordings are also used to ensure patient safety, including with regard to the patient–therapist relationship, added Levine. Corine de Boer, chief medical officer of Multidisciplinary Association for Psychedelic Studies (MAPS) Public Benefit Corporation (PBC), agreed that therapists are important for both safety and efficacy, and with the long duration of treatment sessions, two therapists are essential for practicality and safety. "During psychotherapy outside of the psychedelic world, there is always a power relationship between the therapist and the patient, and psychedelics are no different," she said. Psychedelics may introduce additional risk by creating more openness and more trust, de Boer said.

In addition, the potential for sexual misconduct during treatment sessions has long been a concern to FDA, said Muñiz, in part because of media exposure from specific cases. However, he said this aspect of safety might be beyond the scope of FDA's authority. The agency is working closely with sponsors to discuss specifics about monitoring, video recording, who is in the room, and what degrees and experience the therapists must possess, he said. How this will translate in the real world in terms of cost-effectiveness and delivery burden if these drugs are approved is unknown, said Muñiz.

Set and Setting

Set and setting are considered integral to a positive psychedelic treatment effect, said Muñiz. The regulatory challenges, he said, are (1) identifying the minimum parameters required to ensure safety, and (2) communicating these requirements on the label. He added that the agency is also working with sponsors to protect patients in clinical trials from the "unique risks that may be associated with the nature of these treatments, including sexual misconduct."

Guides or "sitters" are key to ensuring a therapeutic set and setting, yet there are few data to characterize different approaches that sitters may take, said Srinivas Rao, chief scientific officer and co-founder of atai Life Sciences. For example, while many practitioners emphasize the need for a music playlist and eyeshades, he questioned whether there are data to support those elements. He added that the role of sitters is complex and extends beyond the psychedelic experience, reiterating the need for prep work, expectation setting, and support.

Concerns about scaling and standardizing the training and actions of sitters motivated Rao and colleagues to explore digital approaches to standardize therapy. Virtual reality systems could be especially helpful, he said, for example, by enabling the detection of incipient anxiety and modulating it. He suggested that visual stimulation or changing the music might help modulate safety and/or efficacy.

Rao's company is also exploring much shorter acting compounds that could substantially alter the role, or even the need, for a sitter. "Digital may be particularly well suited for some of these compounds," he said.

Minimizing Bias

Sponsors and regulators have also considered various approaches to enable making valid comparisons, minimizing bias, and accounting for the "dramatic functional unblinding," said Muñiz. For psychedelic drug development, the use of traditional placebo controls has significant problems, he said.

Placebo effects, or changes in the neurobiological underpinnings of a clinical outcome, result from positive expectations, prior experience, and other aspects of the therapeutic encounter, such as the patient's mindset, and the psychosocial setting, said Luana Colloca, professor of pain and translational symptom science at the University of Maryland, Baltimore, and an expert in placebo mechanisms. Conditioning can also contribute to the placebo phenomenon, and some people are stronger placebo responders than others (Colloca and Barsky, 2020; Colloca and Miller, 2011). Sanacora added that non-specific effects, or placebo effects, are not unique to psychedelic treatments, but they contribute to a large portion of the effects of most central nervous system treatments.

Some of the strategies researchers have employed include using active controls, subperceptual doses of psychedelics as controls, blinding questionnaires, and raters blinded to the treatment allocation, said Muñiz, noting that each of these approaches has limitations. For example, it may be difficult to identify an active control that has similar subjective effects but is not therapeutic, he said. Low doses of psychedelics may still have psychoactive properties, potentially reducing statistical power and increasing the likelihood of false-negative results. Colloca added that expectations should be measured in both patients and health care providers, and that conditioning can be used to manage placebo effects.

Acknowledging how difficult it is to minimize functional unblinding, Muñiz proposed conducting pivotal dose-response trials without a placebo control, which is explicitly allowed by the Code of Federal Regulations, Title 21, Section 314 and has been addressed in a guidance document from FDA (2003). He said that an NDA could conceivably include just two of these trials but recommended that at least one include a placebo arm for safety characterization.

Additional challenges mentioned by Muñiz include the poorly understood dose-response relationship of psychedelics (Sellers et al., 2018), the generalizability of the treatment given the highly selective patient population enrolled in current studies, the need to understand parameters for retreatment, the need for a non-clinical safety database, and the need for formal studies of abuse potential (Calderon et al., 2018; Sellers et al., 2018). Colloca noted the need for much larger trials than have been conducted thus far, as well as replication studies and data-sharing consortia.

The Role of the Conscious Experience

One remaining unanswered question regarding the critical elements in psychedelic trials is how much the conscious experience has to do with the enduring effects of these drugs, said Sanacora. Charles Raison, the Mary Sue and Mike Shannon Distinguished Chair for Healthy Minds, Children, and Families at the University of Wisconsin–Madison, took the question one step further, asking whether it might be possible to modulate the therapeutic benefit by tweaking the state of consciousness of patients during their psychedelic treatment session.

In Chapter 3, David Olson discussed the development of non-psychedelic psychoplastogens—drugs that have been engineered to remove hallucinogenic-causing properties. If these agents prove to retain therapeutic effects, the implication would be that the conscious psychedelic experience is not necessary, said Raison. Similarly, if people were sedated before taking psychedelics and still experienced relief from their psychiatric symptoms, or even if 1 week or so later they said, "I can't tell you why, but I feel like a different person. I want to live my life differently. I look at the world differently," this too would suggest that the conscious experience is not necessary, said Raison. Blinding trial participants would likely be relatively simple, and such a drug would have enormous commercial appeal, he said. He cautioned, however, that anesthetics might disrupt whatever brain effects were linked to psychedelics and also have antidepressant effects.

Raison suggested that doing those kinds of studies is, from a scientific perspective, one of the most important steps the field needs to take. Moreover, he said that if indeed the conscious experience is not importantly causal, "I think the field has a mandate to figure out what is the least amount of psychosocial support [in which] these agents can be safely administered." Needing less support would improve the cost effectiveness of these treatments and make them easier to scale and standardize, he said.

However, if consciousness is a key player and the narratives that come out of it are driving benefits in some real way, it immediately raises questions about how to optimize the treatment in terms of the depth and longevity of the response, and fully blinding a study would be "more or less logically impossible," said Raison. "We know that unexpected, untoward conscious experiences can produce long-term changes in mental functioning—posttraumatic stress being a classic example of that," he said. "So we would expect to see differential lengths of benefit and hence, differential needs for re-dosing depending on whether or not the conscious experience has causal power or whether it's really more of these basic synaptogenic-type mechanisms."

Raison added that even if the conscious experience is not essential for therapeutic benefits, there might be other potential benefits. He cited a recent 12-month follow-up study of 27 patients treated with psilocybin for moderate to severe depression, in which mystical experiences correlated with increased well-being but did not correlate with persistent antidepressant effects (Gukasyan et al., 2022). "This is an interesting complexity," he said. "Maybe the conscious narrative elements are more impactful on certain relevant metrics than on others." He added that if the conscious experience is not driving efficacy, more frequent re-dosing may be necessary, and relatively similar benefits might be seen both in people who have treatment resistance and in those who are earlier in their disease course. However, if narrative consciousness elements do play a key role, these agents would likely be more impactful early in the disease course or on a recurrent basis in people with treatment-resistant depression, he said.

Sanacora suggested that it is unrealistic to think that the conscious effects are unrelated. "The much harder question is how they are related," he said, and whether other elements that influence the conscious experience, such as set and setting, would need to be optimized individually for each person.

CLINICAL EFFICACY: RECENT TRIALS WITH MDMA AND PSILOCYBIN

Despite the challenges of conducting clinical trials of psychedelics and entactogens, several have been completed or are under way.

MDMA-Assisted Therapy Trials for PTSD

Between 2014 and 2017, MAPS conducted six randomized, double-blind Phase 2 clinical trials of MDMA for the treatment of PTSD, which were reported in a pooled analysis by Mithoefer and colleagues (2019). Collin Reiff, assistant professor of psychiatry at the New York University Grossman School of Medicine, summarized the data from the 105 participants in those trials, who had a mean duration of PTSD of 215.3 months.

Most participants (86.8 percent) had a lifetime history of suicidal ideation and 30.9 percent had a history of suicidal behavior, said Reiff. Prior to starting treatment, there were three non-drug, 90-minute therapy sessions, he said. Approximately two-thirds of the participants received MDMA at doses between 75 and 125 milligrams, while about one-third received a placebo/control dose of 0 to 40 milligrams of MDMA, coupled with manualized psychotherapy in 2- to 3-hour sessions about 1 month apart, said Reiff. Study participants also had three 90-minute, non-drug therapy sessions prior to the first MDMA session, and three to four additional non-drug therapy sessions following each treatment session.

The primary outcome measure was change in total score on the Clinician-Administered PTSD Scale for DSM-IV[2] (CAPS-IV), which was administered at baseline and at follow-up visits. After two blinded experimental sessions, the active group had significantly greater reductions in the CAPS-IV total scores from baseline than the control group, with a Cohen's D effect size of 0.8, which indicates a large treatment effect, said Reiff. Also after two sessions, 54.2 percent of participants in the active group no longer met the DSM-IV PTSD diagnostic criteria compared with 22.6 percent in the control group. Dropout rates were much lower than the average dropout rate for clinical trials, said Reiff.

These Phase 2 trials led to a Phase 3 trial that included 90 adults with chronic PTSD across 15 clinical sites (Mitchell et al., 2021). A CAPS updated with the DSM-5 criteria was used in this trial (CAPS-V), said Reiff. Participants were tapered off their existing medication prior to the study and participated in three preparatory sessions with a male/female therapeutic dyad, followed by an experimental session with MDMA or placebo, and three integration sessions. Each participant received MDMA three times, followed by a set of three integration sessions. In this study, overall scores in CAPS-V dropped nearly 25 points in the MDMA plus psychotherapy group compared with 14 points in the placebo plus psychotherapy group, said Reiff. He added that the MDMA plus psychotherapy group had double the reduction in severity of their PTSD symptoms compared with the placebo group and an effect size of 0.9, "suggesting a large and meaningful difference for MDMA-assisted psychotherapy," said Reiff. As a comparison, he said selective serotonin reuptake inhibitors (SSRIs) approved for the treatment of PTSD have effect sizes between 0.3 and 0.5 in clinical studies.

---

[2] The *Diagnostic and Statistical Manual of Mental Disorders* (DSM) "is the handbook used by health care professionals in the United States and much of the world as the authoritative guide to the diagnosis of mental disorders." The DSM-IV and DSM-5 are earlier editions of the handbook; the DSM-5-TR is the current edition. For more information about the DSM, see https://psychiatry.org/psychiatrists/practice/dsm/frequently-asked-questions (accessed June 12, 2022).

Figure 4-2 graphically illustrates the results of this trial. "The difference for remission is staggering," said Reiff. About 30 percent of participants taking MDMA achieved remission compared with only about 5 percent in the placebo group. He added that MDMA did not induce adverse events of abuse potential, suicidality, or QTc prolongation, a heart condition that can be induced by some drugs.

In 2018, Jerome and colleagues at the MAPS PBC published the results of a pooled analysis of six Phase 2 trials of MDMA-assisted psychotherapy for the treatment of PTSD. The results showed that after two to three active doses of MDMA, there was a reduction in PTSD symptoms within 1 to 2 months of treatment completion and increasing symptom improve-

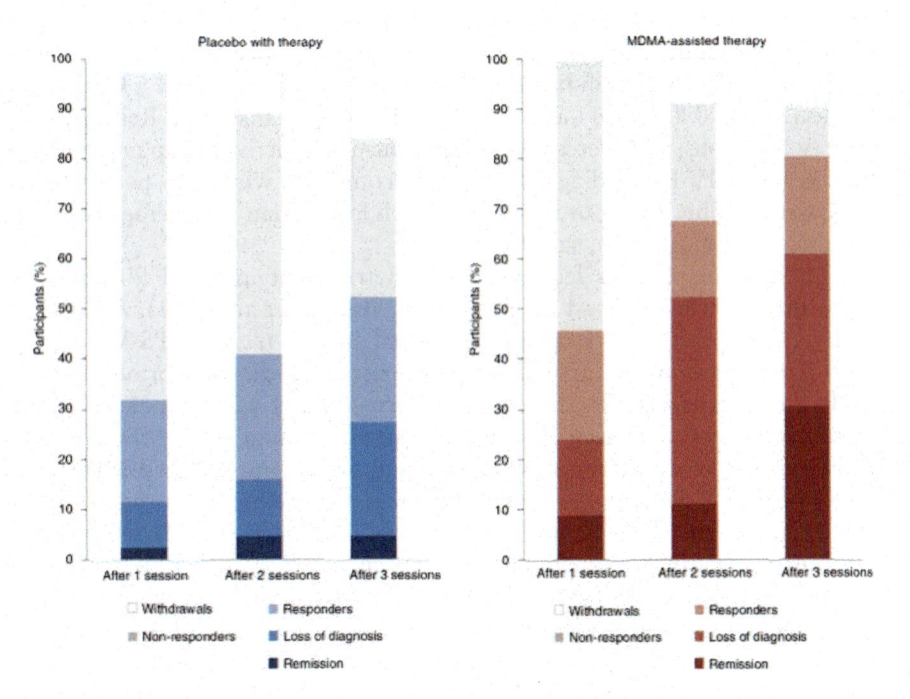

FIGURE 4-2 Treatment response in a Phase 3 trial of MDMA-assisted therapy for PTSD. Response and remission rates as a percentage of total participants randomized to MDMA (red) versus placebo (blue) after each of three treatment sessions. Responders defined as ≥ 10-point decrease in CAPS-V score. Loss of diagnosis defined by specific diagnostic measure on CAPS-V. Remission defined as loss of diagnosis plus a total CAPS-V score of ≤ 11. Non-response defined as a ≤ 10-point decrease on CAPS-V.

NOTE: MDMA = 3,4-methylenedioxymethamphetamine; PTSD = posttraumatic stress disorder.

SOURCES: Presented by Collin Reiff, March 30, 2022; Mitchell et al., 2021.

ment for 12 months (Jerome et al., 2020). The percentage of patients who no longer met PTSD criteria increased by 56 percent at treatment exit to 67 percent at the 12-month follow-up session, according to de Boer. Yet, she noted that MDMA did not work for all participants. Despite having data from 375 patients who were exposed to MDMA in these trials, de Boer said they have not been able to identify prognostic indicators of who will respond to this treatment. "I think this is critical both for the field and for patients and participants," she said. de Boer added that while MDMA is given three times over the course of 4 months, other antidepressants are often given for weeks, months, or years, only to have symptoms return when the medication is stopped.

On the basis of these results, a Phase 3 study was conducted comparing 46 participants who received MDMA to 44 who received the placebo. At the end of the study period, placebo participants were invited to cross over. Long-term data are still being collected, said de Boer. Colloca noted that outcomes observed in crossover designs can be altered by conditioning responses due to prior therapeutic experiences. Response to both placebos and active drugs can be affected by conditioning and learning effects, she said.

In addition to not working for all participants, de Boer said this treatment has clear risks. The Phase 2 study showed that low-dose MDMA does not provide symptom relief and can cause anxiety, she said. Therefore, they used an inactive placebo in the Phase 3 trial. Participants on SSRIs also needed to be tapered off those medications before they could receive MDMA.

de Boer added that increasing diversity among participants and therapists in clinical trials is important. "As we all know, in clinical trials, marginalized communities are underrepresented." Part of the MAPS PBC mission is to make sure these modalities will become available for these communities, she said.

Psilocybin Trials for Depression

Several studies have been reported of the successful use of psilocybin for the treatment of depression and treatment-resistant depression, according to Reiff. In an open-label feasibility trial, 12 participants received two oral doses (10 mg and 25 mg) of psilocybin 7 days apart in a supportive setting, with psychological support provided before, during, and after each session (Carhart-Harris et al., 2016). Depressive symptoms were substantially reduced at week one and at follow-up 3 months later, he said.

This study led to a Phase 2 double-blind, randomized controlled trial comparing psilocybin to the SSRI escitalopram, said Reiff. Patients in the psilocybin group received two doses of 25 milligrams 3 weeks apart, plus 6 weeks of daily placebo (akin to taking escitalopram), while those in the escitalopram group received a 1 milligram dose of psilocybin (control) 3 weeks apart plus 6 weeks of daily oral escitalopram (Carhart-Harris et al., 2021). While this study did not show a significant difference in anti-depressant effects between psilocybin and escitalopram, Reiff said second-ary outcomes "generally favored psilocybin over escitalopram."

In 2019, COMPASS Pathways launched the Phase 2b COMP360 trial to assess the safety, efficacy, and appropriate dosing of psilocybin in partici-pants with treatment-resistant depression. Levine recapped the design and key elements of the trial, in which 233 participants at more than 20 sites in 10 countries received a single dose of an oral synthetic GMP (Good Manu-facturing Practice)-grade formulation of psilocybin. Following preparatory sessions, the treatment was given at one of three doses (1, 10, 25 milligrams) with psychological support from a trained therapist in a standardized, controlled therapeutic setting; integration sessions followed, said Levine. The primary outcome was changed in the Montgomery-Åsperg Depression Rating Scale (MADRS) from baseline to 3 weeks, he said.

Nearly all participants (94 percent) had no prior experience with psychedelics before the trial, said Levine. Two-thirds had a history of sui-cidal thinking or behavior, although candidates with active suicidality were excluded from the trial, he said. He added that participants were withdrawn from other antidepressants before the trial.

Although the results of this study have not been peer reviewed and published, Reiff reported top-line findings that were disseminated by the company through press releases. These reports indicate that the study achieved its primary endpoint with a 25-milligram dose, demonstrating a significant reduction in MADRS score compared with the 1-milligram dose at 1, 3, and 6 weeks after drug administration.

Although the trial used a psychological support model that provided the minimum components of therapy necessary, robust responses were seen with a dose-response relationship, said Levine. A durable effect was seen in a subset of participants, and investigations are under way to understand who responded and who did not, he said.

"This trial is the largest to date and provides a response rate at about one-half of those observed in prior open-label and randomized clinical trials," said Reiff. "This is probably the most explicit evidence we have right now on what treating TRD [treatment-resistant depression] might look like with psilocybin."

Levine also described a separate, small (19-participant), open-label study in which psilocybin was given as an adjunct to an existing SSRI. Although not powered for significance, the study signaled a robust response and remission, said Levine. He called these findings "unexpected" given that there had been preclinical evidence suggesting that chronic adminis-tration of serotonergic antidepressants downregulated the availability of the 5-HT$_{2A}$ receptor as well as anecdotal reports that SSRI antidepressants interfered with the efficacy of psilocybin. Reiff commented that this study suggests that SSRI medication can be taken safely with psilocybin with minimal interference and that COMP360 psilocybin therapy can be taken as a monitored therapy or an adjunctive treatment to SSRI antidepressants.

Levine added that participants in both the 10- and 25-milligram dose groups reported psychedelic experiences. "Also, to some degree that happened with the 1-milligram group," he said. More information on this aspect of the study will be published and presented at upcoming conferences, he said. Reiff suggested that the 1-milligram dose may be similar to what is referred to as a microdose,[3] and could reflect a placebo effect.

Psilocybin Trials for Anxiety and Depression in Patients with Life-Threatening Illness

Patients with life-threatening illnesses, such as cancer, often develop depression and anxiety, which contributes to treatment non-adherence, prolonged hospitalization, increased suicidality, and an overall decreased quality of life (Griffiths et al., 2016). In a double-blind, randomized crossover study of patients with life-threatening cancer and a diagnosis of anxiety or mood disorder, Griffiths and colleagues showed that a high dose (22 or 30 mg) of psilocybin, but not a low dose (1 or 3 mg) (which served as an active control), produced significant decreases in depression and anxiety symptoms after 5 weeks, which persisted through the 6-month follow-up period. A similar double-blind, placebo-controlled randomized crossover study evaluated the efficacy of a single dose of psilocybin combined with psychotherapy in cancer patients with anxiety and depressive symptoms (Ross et al., 2016). This study also demonstrated significant and persistent reductions in all primary measures of depression and anxiety in the psilocybin group compared with the control group.

Psilocybin Trials for Substance Use Disorder

Clinical trials have also demonstrated the effectiveness of psilocybin for treating alcohol use disorder and promoting smoking abstinence, said Reiff. One study enrolled 10 participants who met the DSM-IV criteria for alcohol dependence and had at least 2 heavy drinking days in the previous 30 days. They received 14 sessions of psychotherapy that included motivation enhancement therapy and preparatory sessions, followed by

---

[3] Microdosing with psychedelics was not a topic covered at this workshop. It has not been rigorously studied, according to Raison, nor is there a standard definition for a microdose, said Levine.

two psilocybin-assisted psychotherapy sessions and two debriefing sessions, said Reiff (Bogenschutz et al., 2015). The study demonstrated a significant and sustained increase in abstinence through 36 weeks and has prompted a much larger study by Michael Bogenschutz and his team at New York University that is currently ongoing, he said.

Another study of 15 participants who wanted to quit smoking combined a 15-week course that combined cognitive behavioral therapy with two or three psilocybin treatments, said Reiff (Johnson et al., 2017). At the 6-month follow-up, 80 percent of participants were laboratory verified as abstinent, he said.

5

Anticipating Implementation to Guide Clinical Research and Development

HIGHLIGHTS

- A framework for research and clinical care with respect to psychedelics must address concerns about inequality, equity, and justice (Simon).
- Multiple access dimensions require consideration, including risk factor management, quality and consistency of care, training of a diverse and culturally humble workforce, financial issues such as insurance and reimbursement, social and economic determinants of health, health literacy, stigma, and trust (Simon).
- Ensuring health equity will require strategies to reduce disparities among minoritized and marginalized populations, including people of color, LGBTQIA+ people, and those with physical and sensory disabilities (Dorsen, Simon, Sisti).
- Diversity is critical not only among trial participants and patients, but researchers and clinicians as well (Dudley, Simon).
- Building trust among communities that have been historically marginalized, discriminated against, and treated egregiously will require open, honest communication as the first step toward ensuring equitable access to psychedelic therapy (Dorsen, Dudley, Simon).
- It is important to acknowledge and value Native communities' long history of psychedelic use and how those practices might

increase understanding of the use of psychedelics for the treatment of mental health conditions (Simon).

- Because psychedelic treatment represents a new medical subspecialty, a comprehensive code of ethics that delineates clinical and ethical core competencies and provides clear credentialing and licensing requirements is needed (Sisti).
- Ethical standards, safety guidelines, and enhanced consent procedures are especially needed with regard to therapeutic touch (Sisti).
- A reimbursement structure for psychedelics will be essential to ensure access for people in need, including those of limited means (Levine).
- The off-label and therapeutic use of ketamine and esketamine may provide lessons to guide the implementation of psychedelic therapy (Appelbaum, Levine, Muñiz).
- While the Drug Enforcement Administration has the authority to reschedule psychedelics to a less restrictive designation than Schedule I, there are concerns about the abuse potential of these agents (Coulson).
- The religious or sacramental use of psychedelics may offer valuable lessons about efficacy, delivery, and access (Dorsen).
- Nurses may have a particularly important role to play in the delivery of psychedelic therapy because of their focus on being present for patients and assisting them in many ways through periods of health, illness, and vulnerability (Dorsen).

NOTE: This list is the rapporteurs' summary of points made by the individual speakers identified, and the statements have not been endorsed or verified by the National Academies of Sciences, Engineering, and Medicine. They are not intended to reflect a consensus among workshop participants.

Assuming the efficacy of psychedelics and related compounds is demonstrated for the treatment of mental disorders, the actual benefit derived from implementing these medications in clinical practice is going to depend on a variety of issues, said Paul Appelbaum, the Elizabeth K. Dollard Professor of Psychiatry, Medicine, and Law at the Vagelos College of Physicians and Surgeons at Columbia University. Among these issues is ensuring access and equitable distribution of benefits, especially to people of color and those with limited means, said Appelbaum. Psychedelic treatment may also increase the vulnerability of patients to abuse, he said. There are also questions about how the highly restrictive legal status of these Schedule I drugs,[1] which has hampered research into their clinical effects, may affect the clinical implementation or how the laws may change to enable their use as therapies, said Appelbaum. Other considerations include the potential for abuse and misuse of these medications, off-label prescribing, and commercialization issues.

FRAMEWORKS FOR ACCESSIBLE AND EQUITABLE IMPLEMENTATION

Designing a framework for implementation of research and clinical care that reflects principles of health justice is critical in all areas of health care, but especially with respect to psychedelics, according to Melissa A. Simon, the George H. Gardner Professor of Clinical Gynecology at the Northwestern University Feinberg School of Medicine and the founder and director of both the Center for Health Equity Transformation and the Chicago Cancer Health Equity Collaborative. This framework must address inequality, equity, and justice, she said. Inequality exists when policies or practices favor certain people or groups while actively disadvantaging others, said Simon. Addressing equity requires recognizing that existing policies and practices are inequitable while at the same time providing people with different types of supports that allow them to access their goals despite disadvantages, she added. Finally, Simon said ensuring health justice requires a diverse group of people to evaluate why policies, practices, treatments, and research designs are inequitable.

Acknowledging history is essential in building a health equity and health justice framework, said Simon. "We know that our country has a deep and long history of slavery, racism, and discrimination," she said, including histories of egregious experimentation. Even today, systemic racism limits access of some minoritized and marginalized populations to novel health treatments including psychedelics as well as to clinical trials, said Simon. Not only people of color, but other minoritized populations, such as LGBTQIA+ people, experience significant health disparities compared with heterosexual and cisgender people, added Caroline Dorsen, associate dean of clinical partnerships at the Rutgers University School of Nursing. She added that many of the health care disparities that are especially prominent among LGBTQIA+ people are in the same areas that psychedelics hold promise to address—depression, anxiety, suicidality, and substance

---

[1] According to the U.S. Drug Enforcement Administration (DEA), "Schedule I drugs, substances, or chemicals are defined as drugs with a high potential for abuse, no currently accepted medical use in treatment in the United States, a lack of accepted safety for use under medical supervision." For more information, see https://www.dea.gov/drug-information/drug-scheduling (accessed August 4, 2022).

use disorders. Barriers to accessing psychedelics research studies and care also exist for people with physical disabilities, blindness, hearing impairment, or autism, said Dominic Sisti, assistant professor of medical ethics and health policy at the University of Pennsylvania. He added that people with disabilities also carry a much higher burden of certain mental illnesses that these agents might be able to treat. "We have an ethical obligation to prioritize individuals with disabilities in this research and in practice, but this has not really happened," he said.

Simon noted that the entire research pipeline is fraught with structural racism. Although, Black and Latinx populations represented 13.4 percent and 18.1 percent of the U.S. population in the 2020 census, these populations participate in clinical trials at far lower rates and comprise far lower percentages of U.S. physicians and researchers compared to White people, said Simon. If a study does not have diverse participants, the generalizability of the results may not apply to much of the population, she said. Simon's research team at the Center for Health Equity Transformation has worked with the Health for All Project[2] to better understand how to improve clinical trial participation among minoritized populations. Trust is key, she said. "We have got to work really hard to get back that trust that we severed with our egregious history," said Simon. Dorsen noted, however, that there are few data regarding the participation of LGBTQIA+ people in clinical studies because sexual orientation and gender identity data may not be collected from clinical trial participants.

Diversity among researchers and clinicians is also critical to the impact on—and how connected the research studies are to—minoritized populations, she said. Similarly, "journals, editorial teams, reviewers, and publication opportunities are all fraught with bias," said Simon. "If we are trying to get clinical trials published in key journals, having appropriate editors and reviewers and journal expectations of diverse participation in trials is critical," she added.

Inequities also exist along the entire health care delivery pipeline, said Simon. In developing a framework for accessible and equitable implementation of psychedelic therapy, implementation science is critical, she said. This discipline aims to bridge the science–practice gap using a variety of approaches, including process models, determinant frameworks, and evaluation, she said. In combination with disparities research, implementation science can offer methods and test strategies intended to reduce disparities, said Simon.

Some of the critical access dimensions to consider are risk factor management, quality and consistency of care, training of a diverse and culturally

---

[2] To learn more about the Health for All Project, see https://healthforallproject.org/about (accessed June 4, 2022).

humble workforce, financial issues such as insurance and reimbursement, social and economic determinants of health, health literacy, stigma, and trust, she said. Community health workers and navigators are crucial to building a bridge of trust to the health care system, said Simon. "What is essential to this system working well is care delivery that prioritizes the needs of patients," she said.

BUILDING TRUST WITH MARGINALIZED COMMUNITIES

Charma D. Dudley, vice president of the National Alliance on Mental Illness (NAMI) board of directors and associate director of behavioral health services at Beacon Health Options in Pittsburgh, reinforced the importance of trust. She noted that as a result of the history of Black and Brown people being used for experimental research, and the fact that people of color experience substantial barriers to treatment, "experimental research does not sit well [with them]." When presented the opportunity to receive psychedelics for the treatment of depression, posttraumatic stress disorder (PTSD), or other mental health conditions, Dudley said they may have important questions that need to be answered such as "Is this going to make me crazy?" or "Am I going to lose control?" or "How is this going to help me?"

Medical mistrust may also be a barrier to access in the LGBTQIA+ community, where psychedelics have been used as tools of oppression and possibly as "conversion therapies," added Dorsen.

People do not like to be vulnerable, particularly when they come from a group of people who have experienced oppression, discrimination, and racism on a daily basis, said Dudley. "We need to address the lack of trust in these communities; have open, honest conversations with people regarding psychedelic drugs; and promote awareness," she said.

She added that the Black community is "all about it takes a village." When recommending a course of psychedelic therapy, she suggested allowing them to bring a relative or friend to one of the preparatory sessions, and exposing them to stories of Black and Brown people who have experienced psychedelic therapy would also be helpful, she said. People also want to know that there are people who look like them among the principal investigators and mental health professionals, said Dudley.

Building trust also means educating the community by having researchers go into communities where marginalized people live and talking to ministers, community leaders, activists, and other trusted community members, said Dudley. Simon agreed, noting that every community has different gatekeepers and arbiters of trust. She added that because Native communities have a long history of the use of psychedelics, acknowledging and valuing that history and then linking it to the treatment of mental health conditions is critical.

Intentionally creating inclusive and affirming psychedelic-assisted care for marginalized communities with health disparities, such as LGBTQIA+ people, may be needed, suggested Dorsen. For example, she asked whether processes and protocols exist that speak specifically to the unique culture and health care needs of LGBTQIA+ people. Some protocols call for male/female dyads as therapists, she said, but people who are gender diverse may feel that a binary male/female dyad may not provide the comfort level they need to support a positive therapeutic outcome, she said.

ENSURING SAFE AND ETHICAL RESEARCH AND CARE PRACTICES

As market and social forces quickly propel psychedelics from research to clinical practice, Sisti said a strong ethical scaffold needs to be in place for what is essentially a new medical subspecialty. This would include a comprehensive code of ethics and professionalism, a description of clinical and ethical core competencies, and clear credentialing standards and licensing requirements. Institutional structures are also needed to ensure accountability and sanctions, he said.

Training and credentialing will be required across professions, noted Appelbaum. Even mental health professionals rarely receive the appropriate training, he said. Dorsen noted that the nursing field does not currently have content about psychedelics embedded into its curriculum, although nurses have expertise and experience working with patients in vulnerable moments. She added that some medical schools have initiated collaborative psychedelic psychiatry programs and expressed the hope that nursing schools and schools for other health professions will follow suit. Nurses may have a particularly important role to play in the scalability and delivery of psychedelic therapy because nurses try to "be present for people in illness and in health and see them through vulnerable moments in life," said Dorsen. She suggested there could be roles for many different types of nurses in the psychedelics space, including registered nurses and mental health nurse practitioners who are trained to do psychotherapy as well as doctorally prepared nurses with expertise in quality improvement who can ensure accurate translation of knowledge from clinical trials into the more complicated real-world space.

Steven Levine added that challenges to providing mental health care services are particularly significant in historically underserved communities. Even where professionals are available to deliver needed services, not all of them are reimbursed by Medicare or Medicaid. He said there are active bills looking to potentially expand the reimbursable mental health workforce. There may also be opportunities to expand the mental health workforce through programs like certified peer professionals, although because by definition they would not be trained to deliver psychotherapy or advanced mental health services, the role they would play would need to be defined, said Levine.

Reinforcing what has been previously discussed, Sisti noted that the ethical perils of psychedelic research have been seen throughout its history with egregious examples of unethical research. While psychedelic investigators today must follow a careful regulatory pathway, federal laws, and institutional rules, problems still exist, and there is no consensus about basic ethical questions related to the psychedelic clinical encounter, such as whether it is ever acceptable for researchers or clinicians to touch patients, he said. While some researchers address this question in informed consent and preparatory sessions and try to mitigate the risk through the use of video recording, Sisti said these measures do not always work, resulting in disturbing cases of sexual and psychological abuse in both research and "quasi-underground clinical settings."

He added that certain kinds of touch may be effective and appropriate in therapeutic settings, although even well-intentioned touch may trigger or worsen trauma. To establish broad public trust in this mode of therapy and enable it to be integrated into the health care system, he advocated for harmonizing ethical standards related to touch with the ethical rules for other behavioral health care professionals. As part of the robust U.S. Food and Drug Administration (FDA) risk mitigation program, Sisti suggested establishing safety guidelines and enhanced consent procedures to allow for touch in very specific circumstances. He also suggested screening procedures to "weed out individuals who are ill equipped for these very sensitive patient encounters," for example, individuals drawn to the power of psychedelics and entactogens and the substances' ability to induce suggestibility in an already vulnerable group of individuals. Finally, Sisti said research is needed to identify characteristics of effective therapists in order to filter out the bad apples and provide data for developing evidence-based curricula.

Although patient consent is critical to ensuring safety, Sisti noted several complications. "The consent process itself requires the disclosure of what is essentially ineffable knowledge about the experience that the patient is about to undergo," he said. "That, in and of itself, creates problems in terms of what is the scope of disclosure, how much information you ought to disclose, and what types of information."

Sisti said most researchers use the preparatory session as part of the consent process. They might ask, for example, if the patient would like to be touched if they are struggling with difficult thoughts during the treatment session. However, Sisti noted that sometimes a person will endorse using touch during the preparatory session, yet change their mind during the treatment sessions. "It really boils down to the individual clinician in the moment, drawing on the experience, competency, and wisdom to figure out what is the best choice in that case," he said.

Sisti advocated for an enhanced consent process that helps patients understand what they are about to experience and how it aligns with their values. Through that process, he said, clinicians and researchers may better understand what is appropriate and inappropriate in various situations. Another idea, he said, is to allow family members or other loved ones to be in the room with the patient. Such supportive players would need their own preparation to understand their roles and commit to not being disruptive, said Sisti. Appelbaum added that family members are not always neutral in a person's life, and having them in the room would need to be considered carefully on a case-by-case basis.

Commercialization and Lessons from Ketamine Treatment

Issues around patient access to psychedelics and entactogens were mentioned frequently throughout the workshop. For example, in Chapter 2, in describing her experience receiving methylenedioxymethamphetamine (MDMA) for posttraumatic stress disorder (PTSD), Lori Tipton endorsed the idea of community models of care as a means of reducing barriers that exclude many people in need, especially the historically marginalized. In her remarks, she acknowledged the privilege she has as someone who was able to receive this treatment. She expressed concern about the accessibility of these drugs and therapies, noting that where she lives in New Orleans, many people lack access to basic health care and mental health care. "I have complete faith in the potential of this drug, but I have concerns regarding who will be able to access it in the future," she said.

There are lessons to be learned about the implementation of psychedelic therapy from the off-label and therapeutic use of the anesthetic ketamine and esketamine, which are approved for treating treatment-resistant depression and depression with suicidality, said Levine. While not a psychedelic, ketamine also has psychoactive properties, Levine said. He treated or supervised more than 6,000 patients receiving intravenous ketamine (Levine, 2021). Because this was an off-label use of the drug, it was not reimbursable by payers and therefore unaffordable to many, he said. "There is a paradox that the medicine is cheap, but the delivery is resource intensive and therefore expensive," said Levine.

In 2019, FDA approved esketamine for treatment-resistant depression, with accompanying risk evaluation and mitigation strategy (REMS) and regulated safety standards, which required psychiatrists to be certified to provide this treatment, said Levine. However, he noted that there was no

CPT code[3] and no requirement or means to bill for psychological support, nor was there evidence showing the need for psychological support to ensure safe and efficacious treatment with esketamine. Frustrated psychiatrists quickly reverted to using unregulated racemic ketamine instead, he said.

Looking ahead to upcoming psychedelic therapies should they be approved, Levine said that to achieve broad, safe, and equitable patient access, there will need to be a coding and reimbursement structure in place that is understood by providers and payers and financially viable for them. "In other words, there is a risk that we develop paradigm-shifting new treatments that never get to the patients who may benefit from them and a possible divergence to less regulated routes to access with the accompanying risks or harms," said Levine.

The commercialization of unregulated ketamine led to the proliferation of clinics around the country, added Appelbaum. Some of these clinics are also poised to deliver psychedelic therapy, once it is approved, and may do so with no mental health services or psychotherapeutic component, he said. Levine noted that the approval of esketamine offered some hope of reducing the unregulated use of ketamine. However, lower uptake of esketamine fueled the growth of these less regulated and potentially less safe clinics providing ketamine.

While FDA does not regulate off-label use, including practitioners advertising to the public about providing treatment with psychedelics for specific psychiatric disorders, Javier Muñiz noted that there is an Office of Scientific Investigation within the administration with authority to investigate practices that may fall outside a practitioner's purview. In addition, because these are controlled Schedule I substances, DEA may take action, he said.

NAVIGATING THE LEGAL COMPLEXITY OF MEDICALIZING SCHEDULE I SUBSTANCES

Anthony Coulson, president and owner of NTH Consulting, Inc., and a retired agent of DEA, provided insight into the complicated path to clinical implementation of psychedelics because of their designation as Schedule I substances. In terms of enforcement of laws pertaining to drug use, Coulson said that DEA is essentially a "prohibitionist organization," driven by agents with no training in the field of medicine or scientific research. On the regulatory side, however, they have done a good job of managing the supply of psychedelics in the United States, he said.

---

[3] A Current Procedural Terminology (CPT) code is a medical code established by the American Medical Association to provide uniform language for insurers and health care providers to use when reporting provision of medical services and procedures. To learn more, see https://www.ama-assn.org/practice-management/cpt/cpt-overview-and-code-approval (accessed June 5, 2022).

Coulson said that DEA "defaults to old definitions," for example, using what he considers to be the pejorative word "hallucinogen" rather than psychedelics. The term "hallucinogen" itself is a barrier to research, he said. Yet, he said that while DEA regulations may make it difficult to initiate psychedelics research projects, once a project is given the green light to begin, DEA can be helpful in getting the research done.

Rescheduling a Schedule I agent to a less restrictive designation is within the purview of DEA, yet Coulson said they have no experience in rescheduling psychedelics. They tend to follow the lead of FDA when the research community has persuaded FDA that a drug has a medical benefit. FDA approval triggers DEA consideration of the scheduling designation, he said. However, for DEA, the crux of their decision rests on the drug's abuse potential, said Coulson. Moreover, DEA has the final authority to reschedule a drug unless Congress legislates a change.

Lessons from the Religious and Sacramental Use of Psychedelics

Coulson said that DEA takes a benign enforcement policy to the religious or sacramental use of psychedelics. It is common knowledge that psychedelics are used in these settings, added Dorsen, yet the regulatory and legal issues surrounding these agents make it hard for researchers to learn from the experiences of this community. In particular, these communities could provide potentially valuable lessons related to efficacy, delivery, and access, she said. "People in that community are serious people who are serious about health and healing," said Dorsen. They prioritize emotional and physical safety and have created a system to hold each other accountable as they take these substances to deal with trauma, depression, anxiety, PTSD, and substance abuse, she said. To achieve this, they have incorporated many of the same structures and processes used in clinical trials, such as trained facilitators, music, intention-setting preparatory sessions, and debriefing sessions to make sense of the experience.

Dorsen suggested that these communities could also provide valuable lessons around the practice of delivering psychedelic therapy in group and community settings. This approach could not only increase access and decrease financial burden but may also provide other benefits in terms of reducing the social isolation and lack of connection that may underlie depression, anxiety, and substance abuse. "The group environment, just like group therapy, creates the opportunity for interrelational healing that individual work does not," said Dorsen. She further suggested that as people in these groups begin to see their health in the context of a larger community or culture, there may also be larger benefits to the community.

Dorsen noted that many questions will need to be resolved regarding delivery of psychedelic therapy in group settings, including who is most likely to benefit from a group setting; how should the groups be constituted, for example, would people be grouped on the basis of their life experiences or diagnoses? What sort of preparation and integration would be needed? Would dosing be different because of the interaction of group energy? She suggested that there may also be other unintended benefits from groups, such as increased empathy and decreased bias.

6

Reflecting on the Road Ahead

HIGHLIGHTS

- Psychedelics have the potential to transform psychiatry by providing increased opportunities for amelioration and recovery from psychiatric illnesses (Karlin, Lisanby).
- Knowledge gaps related to clinical efficacy of psychedelics include the reliability, rigor, reproducibility, and generalizability of clinical trials; optimization of both drug and non-drug elements of treatment; mechanism of action; and safety (Lisanby).
- Optimizing safety and ethical parameters during treatment is critical to prevent sexual misconduct by providers while patients are in a vulnerable state (Lisanby).
- While questions remain about the necessity of psychosocial contexts and other non-pharmacological elements, continued research offers opportunities to better understand and potentially incorporate principles such as psychotherapeutic support into other treatment strategies, including traditional pharmacotherapy (Dunn).
- To maximize safety and efficacy, and minimize costs of psychedelic treatment, the separate and combined effects of non-drug treatment elements need to be examined (Gordon).
- Federal agencies need to accelerate the development of knowledge to facilitate translation of positive findings into new

treatments but must resist creating false expectations, which could lead to increased use and/or unintended consequences (Volkow).

- The Food and Drug Administration, Drug Enforcement Administration, and National Institute on Drug Abuse should work together to create mechanisms that enable research to move forward safely on Schedule 1 substances (Volkow).
- Research priorities include better characterization of diverse classes of psychedelic drugs, harmonization of standards, determining how subjective effects may affect therapeutic benefits, and the development of efficacy biomarkers (Dunn, Gordon, Hyman, Volkow).
- NIH clinical and research collaborations with Indigenous populations are important to understand how psychedelic treatment may reduce the impact of trauma (Gordon).
- The Department of Veterans Affairs health system has the potential to be a valuable source of information about the safety and efficacy of psychedelic treatment for trauma-related injuries (Belouin, Dunn).

NOTE: This list is the rapporteurs' summary of points made by the individual speakers identified, and the statements have not been endorsed or verified by the National Academies of Sciences, Engineering, and Medicine. They are not intended to reflect a consensus among workshop participants.

"Exciting and challenging" were the words Sarah H. "Holly" Lisanby, Director of the Division of Translational Research at the National Institute of Mental Health (NIMH), used to summarize the workshop. She said there is tremendous clinical excitement about what could be a "paradigm shift in psychiatric therapeutics" if psychedelics prove to be fast-acting, highly effective, potentially long-lasting treatments for severe major depressive disorder, posttraumatic stress disorder, substance use disorders, and other psychiatric conditions. Neuroscience researchers also expressed great scientific excitement about novel mechanisms that could lead to rapid responses and rapid therapeutic recovery, said Lisanby. "This could be an opportunity to transform our understanding of the neural origins of illness and recovery and development of new treatments that are potentially faster than what we currently have, our existing drugs that take weeks to work," she said. Finally, she said, the societal impact of these agents requires further exploration to avoid some of the mistakes of the past 50 years and ensure responsible use, she said.

CLINICAL CHALLENGES FOR PSYCHEDELIC THERAPY

Data from Phase 2 and 3 clinical trials suggest large effect sizes for the treatment of posttraumatic stress disorder (PTSD) and treatment-resistant depression, and the narratives of individuals who have benefited from psychedelic therapy indicate that psilocybin and 3,4-Methylenedioxymethamphetamine (MDMA) enabled them to live full and rich lives free of the crippling effects of their psychiatric disorders, said Lisanby. Yet, she noted that several challenges remain.

The first concern, she said, is the reliability of the reported large effect sizes, which could have been influenced by bias; unblinding of patients, therapists, and raters; patients' and therapists' expectations about the benefits of the therapy; placebo effects; and conditioning, which could confound crossover trial designs. Alternative trial designs, such as using active comparators, objective outcome measures, and biomarkers, could help mitigate these challenges, said Lisanby. She also raised concerns about the rigor, reproducibility, and generalizability of these trials, particularly because they were conducted mostly with relatively small sample sizes in self-selected groups of participants and typically exclude people with a history of psychosis or suicide attempts. "This limits knowledge about outcomes in diverse patient groups," she said.

Related to clinical efficacy, Lisanby mentioned significant knowledge gaps, including the importance of and optimal format for the psychotherapeutic component of treatment, whether the subjective hallucinogenic experience is required to achieve efficacy, the mechanisms of action of these agents, the interindividual variability in response, and safety concerns about the drug itself and the psychosocial context in which the drugs are used. One of the questions about drug safety is whether the powerful neuroplasticity effects could be maladaptive, she said. There are also risks of cardiotoxicity and aversive experiences during treatment, as well as unanswered questions about the abuse potential of these agents, said Lisanby. Safety concerns have also been raised related to the risk of boundary violations and sexual misconduct by providers while patients are in a vulnerable state, she said.

Implementing clinical therapy with psychedelics poses further challenges related to optimal dosing and standardization of provider and therapist training, she said. Dose-response studies that address both the optimal dose range of the drug and the psychotherapy are currently lacking, said Lisanby. Questions also remain about the long-term durability of treatment effects and the minimum amount of psychosocial support needed, which goes to the question of scalability, she said, adding that group therapy sessions could potentially address some of the scalability concerns.

Scientific Impact and Remaining Challenges

An emerging literature base in both humans and animal studies has begun to shed light on the molecular, cellular, and circuit-level mechanisms in different brain regions that underlie the effects of psychedelics, noted Lisanby. Even when the psychogenic and hallucinogenic properties of psychedelics are removed through chemical modifications, structural and functional plasticity and increased dendritic spine growth remain and might mediate therapeutic benefits, though this has yet to be tested in humans she said.

The testimonies of Nora Osowski and Lori Tipton in Chapter 2 emphasized the important role played by therapists during, before, and after drug administration. They cited the meaning they derived from the therapeutic experience as a factor essential to them receiving a beneficial treatment effect. While set and setting continue to be considered essential non-drug elements of psychedelic therapy, evidence on the mechanisms underlying those processes is only correlational at this point, said Lisanby.

Lisanby cited several scientific challenges that can only be answered through additional research. "We need to know more across the board," she said, from molecular to psychological levels, to understand what is necessary and sufficient to achieve efficacy and ensure safety, she said.

Psychedelics' Societal Impact: From Counterculture to Therapy

In Chapter 2, Charles Grob described the long history of psychedelics, dating back thousands of years to shamanic cultures and Indigenous peoples. Lisanby noted that as Western medical communities began to explore therapeutic applications of these agents in the 1960s, they seeped out of the medical arena and into the "counterculture movement." Now, as the medical and scientific communities are again looking toward these compounds as therapeutic interventions, steps are needed to ensure that society is ready for responsible use of these agents, she said. She called for a consensus on terminology and classification of these drugs; an industry ecosystem to develop pharmaceutical grade compounds for research; professional and ethical standards around the conduct and safety monitoring of these agents; methods of accountability around the use of therapeutic touch to protect from boundary violations; and the use of an enhanced consent process to better inform patients of risks and benefits.

To generate safety and efficacy data that will support FDA approval, large, adequately powered, and well-controlled trials are needed, and for both these trials and future clinical treatment, equitable access to diverse communities is essential, said Lisanby. As noted by Charma D. Dudley, Caroline Dorsen, and Dominic Sisti, this will require developing trust across diverse communities, such as people of color, LGBTQIA+, and people with disabilities, as well as diverse representation among researchers and across all members of interprofessional care teams.

PERSPECTIVES FROM A DIVERSE GROUP OF STAKEHOLDERS

Given the emerging themes as summarized in this chapter, a panel of stakeholders from industry, academia, the federal government, and patient advocacy groups was convened to discuss critical research gaps, potential next steps, and promising opportunities for future action.

The Promise and Peril of Psychedelics

Daniel Karlin, chief medical officer at MindMed, cited both the promise and the peril of psychedelic drugs. The promise would be realized if these drugs lead the field to "return to a psychiatry that is oriented toward cure and recovery" rather than accepting moderate-effect sizes and treatments that help some of the people some of the time, said Karlin. The peril, he said, is that the field fails to get these drugs to people in a reasonable and safe way. "We absolutely have to ensure that there are systems in place so that the folks most in need, the folks left behind by society, are able to access these drugs and get their benefits."

From the perspective of the federal government, and the Substance Abuse and Mental Health Services Administration (SAMHSA) in particular, the field around psychedelics is currently faced with a unique opportunity, as more people are coming into the field and paying attention to the complex and crucial issues that need to be addressed, said Captain Sean Belouin, a clinical pharmacist with the U.S. Public Health Service. SAMHSA wants to ensure that the best science is guiding decision making and that the use of psychedelics is done responsibly, accountably, safely, and ethically to prevent misuse, he said. He added that preventing misuse is foundational to harm reduction, risk mitigation, and safety monitoring.

Determining the Necessity of Multiple Treatment Elements

Walter Dunn provided the perspective of a clinical trialist, researcher, and clinician. He is an assistant professor of psychiatry at the University of California, Los Angeles, and section chief for mood disorders at the Greater Los Angeles Veterans Affairs Healthcare system. Dunn suggested that it may not be possible to arrive at a point where the elements of treatment can be strictly divided into those that are essential and those that are not. "I think the answer will be, 'it depends,'" he said. There will be clinical situations where two therapists and 6 hours of preparation are essential for safety and efficacy, and other situations where one therapist and an hour of preparation will suffice, said Dunn. Rather than a single, one-size-fits-all approach, Dunn envisions multiple validated and well-studied permutations of a treatment model that can be adapted to a diversity of clinical situations.

Dunn further suggested that rather than talking about how these treatment paradigms can be stripped down to make them fit within a broken medical system, the field should be learning from the experiences of psychedelic-assisted therapy and incorporate principles such as psychotherapeutic support into other treatment strategies. "Perhaps it is the therapeutic alliance and the time spent understanding our patients that is at the crux of why these treatments work so well," he said. To that end, he noted that the real-world application of these treatments in all of their permutations and in a complex patient population provides tremendous learning opportunities for both clinicians and policy makers.

However, Joshua Gordon, director of National Institute of Mental Health (NIMH), said that while there is not good evidence for the need for the different components, there are "good, inherent, moral imperatives" to describe the relative efficacy of each of these components because of safety and availability issues as well as costs to both the patient and the system. There is a moral imperative to study the separate and conjoint effects of these various aspects, he said.

Dunn added that there may also be other psychotherapeutic modalities that combined with psychedelics could achieve similar levels of efficacy and safety. He noted that the types of psychotherapies currently used in the Multidisciplinary Association for Psychedelic Studies (MAPS) or COMPASS protocols may limit the rollout if their approvals specify that treatment is limited to clinicians trained in these specific psychotherapy models. Most clinicians have not been formally trained in the MAPS or COMPASS therapy models, although they are likely to be trained in other therapy modalities, such as cognitive behavioral therapy.

Nora Volkow added that what may be valid for one indication may not necessarily be valid for another. "We have to be more specific in our language," she said. For example, she said one of the things that happens in addiction is that a person loses the capacity for self-regulation. A mechanism that improves self-regulation, even if it does not affect other neurocircuits, could improve the likelihood of successful recovery in individuals treated for substance use disorder, said Volkow. For other mental illnesses, she suggested determining to what extent targeting certain neurocircuits could be beneficial without necessarily affecting all elements of the experience.

Advancing High-Quality Research

Psychedelics offer hope for a better future for people with mental illness, but their potential will only be realized with more high-quality research, said Shirley Holloway, president of the National Alliance on Mental Illness (NAMI) board of directors. Holloway also endorsed Charles Raison's call for early intervention. Yet, public perception will play a crucial role in the future use of psychedelics, she said, recalling Thomas Insel and Paul Summergrad's admonition at the 2017 Psychedelic Science conference that a "single, sloppy, researcher or patient with a disastrous experience would poison the well for everybody."

Volkow agreed that federal agencies need to accelerate the development of knowledge that can facilitate that translation of "very tantalizing" findings into potential treatments for mental illness; however, she cautioned about losing perspective and creating expectations that are too high, which can lead to increased use. "We have seen that happen with the promise of marijuana as a potential therapeutic for a wide variety of diseases and disorders," she said.

In terms of research priorities, Volkow said there are some "low-hanging fruits," such as better characterization of diverse types of drugs that are called psychedelics. She noted that during the COVID-19 pandemic, harmonization of standards emerged as a valuable endeavor and suggested that there are ways to achieve standardization while still allowing flexibility. A major obstacle that slowed down cannabis research and is also likely to slow down psychedelic research was the scaling process, she said. In addition, working with both the Food and Drug Administration (FDA) and Drug Enforcement Administration (DEA) will be essential to enable research to move forward on Schedule I substances without having to go through the procedures that are intended for non-research-related drug users. She added that as the director of National Institute on Drug Abuse (NIDA), she cannot ignore the potential of psychedelics for misuse and the need to minimize adverse consequences.

Gordon said that for safety reasons, the most important and controversial question is whether the subjective effects are required for therapeutic action. He acknowledged that there are powerful arguments in support of the hypothesis that subjective effects are inextricably linked to the therapeutic action via neuroplastic effects. "I think it's a hypothesis we need to test," he said. Indeed, he added, "there is no such thing as experience without neurobiology." Even if subjective experiences are essential for treatment effects, those subjective effects are driven by neurobiology, he said.

In support of the idea that subjective experience may be essential, Dunn offered the disease model of posttraumatic stress disorder (PTSD) to highlight the critical role of subjective experience in driving neurobiological changes and the resulting symptomology and functional impairment. In PTSD, the traumatic event is wholly a subjective distressing experience that is the necessary precipitant leading to a distorted or negative narrative that persists and contributes to depression and patient functional impairment. He suggested that an intense positive valence experience, such as those induced by psychedelics or entactogens, could function in a similar capacity but yield a durable positive narrative that could facilitate recovery from psychiatric illness and improved resilience to future stressors. Investigator-initiated research is critical, said Karlin, but can be hampered by regulations and lack of access to research-grade psychedelic agents. Volkow noted that researchers can obtain Schedule I substances from NIDA and other suppliers, as long as those sources are approved by the DEA. Schedule 1 substances can also be imported from other countries with appropriate DEA approvals, she said.

Promoting Diversity and Ensuring Equity in Research and Care

Volkow reinforced what many other workshop participants have discussed about the need to recruit diverse populations for clinical trials, adding that this will require addressing the unique challenges posed by some minority and underserved groups, including the lack of trust in governmental organizations and health care systems. She added that the economics of these agents should also be incorporated into research models to ensure that these treatments are accessible, equitable, and sustainable. Finally, she suggested that lack of trust may influence the psychedelic experience itself and said this possibility will need to be investigated.

Lisanby noted that, as has been previously discussed in terms of health care justice and equity, trauma runs deep in Indigenous communities, and it is particularly important not to leave these populations behind in the development of psychedelics and entactogens. The challenge, said Holloway, is how to provide high-quality treatment to Indigenous communities. The trauma in these groups has many layers, she said. "It is just layer after layer of issues that need to be addressed in a very thoughtful way, with cultural humility," she said.

Gordon said the National Institutes of Health (NIH) has several clinical and translational research collaborations with tribal nations and in Alaskan, Indian, and Native American populations in the United States, and is open to other ideas for understanding the use of psychedelic treatments for reducing the impact of trauma in these populations.

Addressing the Mental Health Needs of Military Service Members

Many veterans have suffered serious trauma and moral injury associated with combat, and current therapies are not addressing their needs, said Belouin. He suggested that psychedelics could be used as part of the biopsychosocial spiritual therapy model, which is used across all hospitals and hospice palliative care networks to treat patients with existential distress and demoralization. This model, he said, involves the entire spectrum of clinical and non-clinical health care practitioners trained in counseling, including physicians, nurses, pharmacists, social workers, licensed counselors, and faith-based practitioners. He encouraged people working in the psychedelic field to broaden their minds in terms of the types of individuals who can support patients receiving treatment. It will require a significant workforce, with interdisciplinary cross-training, credentialing, and licensing, he said.

Dunn added that much of the movement and energy to advance research into psychedelic-assisted therapy has come from veterans, working behind the scenes to influence state legislatures to increase funding in this area. As an integrated health care system, the Department of Veterans Affairs (VA) system also has the potential to be a valuable source of information about safety and efficacy when these treatments are rolled out clinically, said Dunn. He noted that the VA was able to roll out esketamine soon after its approval, getting this new treatment to veterans quickly with an enhanced risk evaluation and mitigation strategy (REMS)–like program, safety parameters, and the systematic collection of data on safety and efficacy. Other managed health care systems could also potentially collect high-level quality data if they choose to roll out novel treatments soon after approval, he said.

The Search for Biomarkers

Given the challenge of confirming efficacy in the absence of placebo controls or other comparators, during the open discussion, Steven Hyman, director of the Stanley Center for Psychiatric Research at the Broad Institute of Harvard and Massachusetts Institute of Technology (MIT), suggested that objective efficacy biomarkers might provide a solution. Positron emission tomography (PET) binding of serotonin receptors is clearly a mechanistic biomarker for target engagement, he said, but has not been used as an efficacy biomarker. Volkow noted that PET can also be used to assess receptor occupancy to guide dosing and timing. She added that functional magnetic resonance imagining (fMRI) can provide information regarding a drug's effect on circuitry, which can be used to predict a response. Because this methodology may be useful in detecting an early signal and for assessing the differences in responses among individuals, she suggested that fMRI may provide an indicator of treatment success.

Lisanby added that FDA has begun to emphasize the importance of patient-reported outcomes in the regulatory pathway. "It is not a biomarker per se, but is something that transcends diagnosis and really looks at whether [a treatment] is making a difference in the person's life," she said. Indeed, said Karlin, because psychiatric illnesses such as major depressive disorder are subjectively defined with no meaningful biological construct, the only way to know what a person is feeling is to ask them.

One potential early "objective" marker of response might be objective changes or subjective improvement in sleep, added Dunn. He said this has been observed in patients who responded to treatment with selective serotonin reuptake inhibitors (SSRIs).

CONCLUDING REMARKS

Sanacora concluded the workshop by reiterating the excitement, optimism, and promise of psychedelics, balancing this against concerns about the complexity, ethics, licensing, regulatory oversight, public health, and health equity issues that need resolution. "The workshop provided a solid platform to launch us into the next phase of research and development in this area," he said.

A

References

Barrett, F. S., M. K. Doss, N. D. Sepeda, J. J. Pekar, and R. R. Griffiths. 2020. Emotions and brain function are altered up to one month after a single high dose of psilocybin. *Scientific Reports* 10(1):2214. https://doi.org/10.1038/s41598-020-59282-y.

Bender, D., and D. J. Hellerstein. 2022. Assessing the risk–benefit profile of classical psychedelics: A clinical review of second-wave psychedelic research. *Psychopharmacology* 239:1907–1932. https://doi.org/10.1007/s00213-021-06049-6.

Bogenschutz, M. P., A. A. Forcehimes, J. A. Pommy, C. E. Wilcox, P. C. R. Barbosa, and R. J. Strassman. 2015. Psilocybin-assisted treatment for alcohol dependence: A proof-of-concept study. *Journal of Psychopharmacology* 29(3):289–299. https://doi.org/10.1177/0269881114565144.

Calderon, S. N., J. Hunt, and M. Klein. 2018. A regulatory perspective on the evaluation of hallucinogen drugs for human use. *Neuropharmacology* 142(November):135–142. https://doi.org/10.1016/j.neuropharm.2017.11.028.

Cameron, L. P., R. J. Tombari, J. Lu, A. J. Pell, Z. Q. Hurley, Y. Ehinger, M. V. Vargas, M. N. McCarroll, J. C. Taylor, D. Myers-Turnbull, T. Liu, B. Yaghoobi, L. J. Laskowski, E. I. Anderson, G. Zhang, J. Viswanathan, B. M. Brown, M. Tija, L. E. Dunlap, Z. T. Rabow, O. Fiehn, H. Wulff, J. D. McCorvy, P. J. Lein, D. Kokel, D. Ron, J. Peters, Y. Zuo, and D. E. Olson. 2021. A non-hallucinogenic psychedelic analogue with therapeutic potential. *Nature* 589(7842):474–479. https://doi.org/10.1038/s41586-020-3008-z.

Carhart-Harris, R. L., M. Bolstridge, J. Rucker, C. M. J. Day, D. Erritzoe, M. Kaelen, M. Bloomfield, J. A. Rickard, B. Forbes, A. Feilding, D. Taylor, S. Pilling, V. Curran, and D. J. Nutt. 2016. Psilocybin with psychological support for treatment-resistant depression: An open-label feasibility study. *The Lancet Psychiatry* 3(7):619–627. https://doi.org/10.1016/S2215-0366(16)30065-7.

Carhart-Harris, R. L., L. Roseman, E. Haijen, D. Erritzoe, R. Watts, I. Branchi, and M. Kaelen. 2018. Psychedelics and the essential importance of context. *Journal of Psychopharmacology* 32(7):725–731. https://doi.org/10.1177/0269881118754710.

Carhart-Harris, R., B. Giribaldi, R. Watts, M. Baker-Jones, A. Murphy-Beiner, R. Murphy, J. Martell, A. Blemings, D. Erritzoe, and D. J. Nutt. 2021. Trial of psilocybin versus escitalopram for depression. *New England Journal of Medicine* 384(15):1402–1411. https://doi.org/10.1056/NEJMoa2032994.

Colloca, L., and A. J. Barsky. 2020. Placebo and nocebo effects. *New England Journal of Medicine* 382(6):554–561. https://doi.org/10.1056/NEJMra1907805.

Colloca, L., and F. G. Miller. 2011. How placebo responses are formed: A learning perspective. *Philosophical Transactions of the Royal Society B: Biological Sciences* 366(1572):1859–1869. https://doi.org/10.1098/rstb.2010.0398.

Corkery J. M. 2018. Ibogaine as a treatment for substance misuse: Potential benefits and practical dangers. *Progress in Brain Research* 242:217–257. https://doi.org/10.1016/bs.pbr.2018.08.005.

De Gregorio, D., A. Aguilar-Valles, K. H. Preller, B. D. Heifets, M. Hibicke, J. Mitchell, and G. Gobbi. 2021a. Hallucinogens in mental health: Preclinical and clinical studies on LSD, psilocybin, MDMA, and ketamine. *Journal of Neuroscience* 41(5):891–900.

De Gregorio, D., J. Popic, J. P. Enns, A. Inserra, A. Skalecka, A. Markopoulos, L. Posa, M. Lopez-Canul, H. Qianzi, C. K. Lafferty, J. P. Britt, S. Comai, A. Aguilar-Valles, N. Sonenberg, and G. Gobbi. 2021b. Lysergic acid diethylamide (LSD) promotes social behavior through MTORC1 in the excitatory neurotransmission. *Proceedings of the National Academy of Sciences of the United States of America* 118(5):e2020705118. https://doi.org/10.1073/pnas.2020705118.

De Gregorio, D., A. Inserra, J. P. Enns, A. Markopoulos, M. Pileggi, Y. El Rahimy, M. Lopez-Canul, S. Comai, and G. Gobbi. 2022. Repeated lysergic acid diethylamide (LSD) reverses stress-induced anxiety-like behavior, cortical synaptogenesis deficits and serotonergic neurotransmission decline. *Neuropsychopharmacology* 47(6):1188–1198. https://doi.org/10.1038/s41386-022-01301-9.

Dolder, P. C., Y. Schmid, F. Müller, S. Borgwardt, and M. E. Liechti. 2016. LSD acutely impairs fear recognition and enhances emotional empathy and sociality. *Neuropsychopharmacology* 41(11):2638–2646. https://doi.org/10.1038/npp.2016.82.

Droogmans, S., B. Cosyns, H. D'haenen, E. Creeten, C. Weytjens, P. R. Franken, B. Scott, D. Schoors, A. Kemdem, L. Close, and J. L. Vandenbossche. 2007. Possible association between 3, 4-methylenedioxymethamphetamine abuse and valvular heart disease. *The American Journal of Cardiology* 100(9):1442–1445.

FDA (Food and Drug Administration). 2003. Guidance for industry: Exposure–response relationship—study design, data analysis, and regulatory applications. Department of Health and Human Services. https://www.fda.gov/media/71277/download.

Gasser, P., K. Kirchner, and T. Passie. 2015. LSD-assisted psychotherapy for anxiety associated with a life-threatening disease: A qualitative study of acute and sustained subjective effects. *Journal of Psychopharmacology* 29(1):57–68. https://doi.org/10.1177/0269881114555249.

GBD (Global Burden of Disease) 2019 Mental Disorders Collaborators. 2022. Global, regional, and national burden of 12 mental disorders in 204 countries and territories, 1990–2019: A systematic analysis for the global burden of disease study 2019. *The Lancet Psychiatry* 9(2):137–150. https://doi.org/10.1016/S2215-0366(21)00395-3.

Griffiths, R. R., M. W. Johnson, M. A. Carducci, A. Umbricht, W. A. Richards, B. D. Richards, M. P. Cosimano, and M. A. Klinedinst. 2016. Psilocybin produces substantial and sustained decreases in depression and anxiety in patients with life-threatening cancer: A randomized double-blind trial. *Journal of Psychopharmacology* 30(12):1181–1197. https://doi.org/10.1177/0269881116675513.

Grinspoon, L., and J. B. Bakalar. 1979. Psychedelic drugs reconsidered. Vol. 168. New York: Basic Books.

Grob, C. S., R. E. Poland, L. Chang, and T. Ernst. 1996. Psychobiologic effects of 3,4 -methylenedioxymethamphetamine in humans: Methodological considerations and preliminary observations. *Behavioural Brain Research* 73(1–2):103–107. https://doi.org/10.1016/0166-4328(96)00078-2.

Gukasyan, N., A. K. Davis, F. S. Barrett, M. P. Cosimano, N. D. Sepeda, M. W. Johnson, and R. R. Griffiths. 2022. Efficacy and safety of psilocybin-assisted treatment for major depressive disorder: Prospective 12-month follow-up. *Journal of Psychopharmacology* 36(2):151–158. https://doi.org/10.1177/02698811211073759.

Hayes, S. C., K. D. Strosahl, and K. G. Wilson. 1999. *Acceptance and commitment therapy an experiential approach to behavior change.* New York: Guilford Press.

Holmes, S. E., S. J. Finnema, M. Naganawa, N. DellaGioia, D. Holden, K. Fowles, M. Davis, J. Ropchan, P. Emory, Y. Ye, N. Nabulsi, D. Matuskey, G. A. Angarita, R. H. Pietrzak, R. S. Duman, G. Sanacora, J. H. Krystal, R. E. Carson, and I. Esterlis. 2022. Imaging the effect of ketamine on synaptic density (SV2A) in the living brain. *Molecular Psychiatry* 27(4):2273–2281. https://doi.org/10.1038/s41380-022-01465-2.

Inserra, A., D. De Gregorio, T. Rezai, M. G. Lopez-Canul, S. Comai, and G. Gobbi. 2021. Lysergic acid diethylamide differentially modulates the reticular thalamus, mediodorsal thalamus, and infralimbic prefrontal cortex: An in vivo electrophysiology study in male mice. *Journal of Psychopharmacology* 35(4):469–482. https://doi.org/10.1177/0269881121991569.

Jerome, L., A. A. Feduccia, J. B. Wang, S. Hamilton, B. Yazar-Klosinski, A. Emerson, M. C. Mithoefer, and R. Doblin. 2020. Long-term follow-up outcomes of MDMA-assisted psychotherapy for treatment of PTSD: A longitudinal pooled analysis of six phase 2 trials. *Psychopharmacology* 237(8):2485–2497. https://doi.org/10.1007/s00213-020-05548-2.

Johnson, M. W., A. Garcia-Romeu, and R. R. Griffiths. 2017. Long-term follow-up of psilocybin-facilitated smoking cessation. *The American Journal of Drug and Alcohol Abuse* 43(1):55–60. https://doi.org/10.3109/00952990.2016.1170135.

Johnson, M. W., R. R. Griffiths, P. S. Hendricks, and J. E. Henningfield. 2018. The abuse potential of medical psilocybin according to the 8 factors of the Controlled Substances Act. *Neuropharmacology* 142:143–166. https://doi.org/10.1016/j.neuropharm.2018.05.012.

Kettner, H., F. E. Rosas, C. Timmermann, L. Kärtner, R. L. Carhart-Harris, and L. Roseman. 2021. Psychedelic communitas: Intersubjective experience during psychedelic group sessions predicts enduring changes in psychological wellbeing and social connectedness. *Frontiers in Pharmacology* 12. https://www.frontiersin.org/article/10.3389/fphar.2021.623985.

Kyzar, E. J., C. D. Nichols, R. R. Gainetdinov, D. E. Nichols, and A. V. Kalueff. 2017. Psychedelic drugs in biomedicine. *Trends in Pharmacological Sciences* 38(11):992–1005. https://doi.org/10.1016/j.tips.2017.08.003.

Levine, S. 2021. Ketamine: A cautionary tale. *Psychology Today.* https://www.psychologytoday.com/us/blog/pathways-progress/202111/ketamine-cautionary-tale.

Ly, C., A. C. Greb, L. P. Cameron, J. M. Wong, E. V. Barragan, P. C. Wilson, K. F. Burbach, S. Soltanzadeh, S. S. Zarandi, A. Sood, M. R. Paddy, and W. C. Duim. 2018. Psychedelics promote structural and functional neural plasticity. *Cell Reports* 23(11):3170–3182. https://doi.org/10.1016/j.celrep.2018.05.022.

Markopoulos, A., A. Inserra, D. De Gregorio, and G. Gobbi. 2021. Evaluating the potential use of serotonergic psychedelics in autism spectrum disorder. *Frontiers in Pharmacology* 12.

McCulloch, D. E.-Wen, M. K. Madsen, D. S. Stenbæk, S. Kristiansen, B. Ozenne, P. S. Jensen, G. M. Knudsen, and P. M. Fisher. 2022. Lasting effects of a single psilocybin dose on resting-state functional connectivity in healthy individuals. *Journal of Psychopharmacology* 36(1):74–84. https://doi.org/10.1177/02698811211026454.

Mitchell, J. M., M. Bogenschutz, A. Lilienstein, C. Harrison, S. Kleiman, K. Parker-Guilbert, M. Ot'alora G, W. Garas, C. Paleos, I. Garman, C. Nicholas, M. Mithoefer, S. Carlin, B. Poulter, A. Mithoefer, S. Quevedo, G. Wells, S. S. Klaire, B. van der Kolk, K. Tzarfaty, R. Amiaz, R. Worthy, S. Shannon, J. D. Woolley, C. Marta, Y. Gelfand, E. Hapke, S. Amar, Y. Wallach, R. Brown, S. Hamilton, J. B. Wang, A. Coker, R. Matthews, A. de Boer, B. Yazar-Klosinski, A. Emerson, and R. Doblin. 2021. MDMA-assisted therapy for severe PTSD: A randomized, double-blind, placebo-controlled phase 3 study. *Nature Medicine* 27(6):1025–1033. https://doi.org/10.1038/s41591-021-01336-3.

Mithoefer, M. C., A. A. Feduccia, L. Jerome, A. Mithoefer, M. Wagner, Z. Walsh, S. Hamilton, B. Yazar-Klosinski, A. Emerson, and R. Doblin. 2019. MDMA-assisted psychotherapy for treatment of PTSD: Study design and rationale for phase 3 trials based on pooled analysis of six phase 2 randomized controlled trials. *Psychopharmacology* 236(9):2735–2745. https://doi.org/10.1007/s00213-019-05249-5.

Nichols, D. E. 2022. Entactogens: How the name for a novel class of psychoactive agents originated. *Frontiers in Psychiatry* 13. https://www.frontiersin.org/article/10.3389/fpsyt.2022.863088.

Pahnke, W. N., and W. A. Richards. 1966. Implications of LSD and experimental mysticism. *Journal of Religion and Health* 5(3):175–208. https://doi.org/10.1007/BF01532646.

Petranker, R., T. Anderson, and N. Farb. 2020. Psychedelic research and the need for transparency: Polishing Alice's looking glass. *Frontiers in Psychology* 11:1681. https://doi.org/10.3389/fpsyg.2020.01681.

Preller, K. H., A. Razi, P. Zeidman, P. Stämpfli, K. J. Friston, and F. X. Vollenweider. 2019. Effective connectivity changes in LSD-induced altered states of consciousness in humans. *Proceedings of the National Academy of Sciences of the United States of America* 116(7):2743–2748. https://doi.org/10.1073/pnas.1815129116.

Reiff, C. M., E. E. Richman, C. B. Nemeroff, L. L. Carpenter, A. S. Widge, C. I. Rodriguez, N. H. Kalin, W. M. McDonald, and the Work Group on Biomarkers and Novel Treatments, a Division of the American Psychiatric Association Council of Research. 2020. Psychedelics and psychedelic-assisted psychotherapy. *American Journal of Psychiatry* 177(5):391–410. https://doi.org/10.1176/appi.ajp.2019.19010035.

Roseman, L., D. J. Nutt, and R. L. Carhart-Harris. 2018. Quality of acute psychedelic experience predicts therapeutic efficacy of psilocybin for treatment-resistant depression. *Frontiers in Pharmacology* 8. https://www.frontiersin.org/article/10.3389/fphar.2017.00974.

Roseman, L., E. Haijen, K. Idialu-Ikato, M. Kaelen, R. Watts, and R. Carhart-Harris. 2019. Emotional breakthrough and psychedelics: Validation of the emotional breakthrough inventory. *Journal of Psychopharmacology* 33(9):1076–1087. https://doi.org/10.1177/0269881119855974.

Ross, S., A. Bossis, J. Guss, G. Agin-Liebes, T. Malone, B. Cohen, S. E. Mennenga, A. Belser, K. Kalliontzi, J. Babb, Z. Su, P. Corby, and B. Schmidt. 2016. Rapid and sustained symptom reduction following psilocybin treatment for anxiety and depression in patients with life-threatening cancer: A randomized controlled trial. *Journal of Psychopharmacology* 30(12):1165–1180. https://doi.org/10.1177/0269881116675512.

Rucker, J. J., L. Marwood, R.-L. J. Ajantaival, C. Bird, H. Eriksson, J. Harrison, M. Lennard-Jones, S. Mistry, F. Saldarini, S. Stansfield, S. J. Tai, S. Williams, N. Weston, E. Malievskaia, and A. H. Young. 2022. The effects of psilocybin on cognitive and emotional functions in healthy participants: Results from a phase 1, randomised, placebo-controlled trial involving simultaneous psilocybin administration and preparation. *Journal of Psychopharmacology* 36(1):114–125. https://doi.org/10.1177/02698811211064720.

Schulenberg, J. E., M. E. Patrick, L. D. Johnston, P. M. O'Malley, J. G. Bachman, and R. A. Miech. 2021. Monitoring the Future national survey results on drug use, 1975–2020: Volume II, College students and adults ages 19–60. Ann Arbor, MI: Institute for Social Research, University of Michigan. http://monitoringthefuture.org/pubs.html#monographs.

Sellers, E. M., M. K. Romach, and D. B. Leiderman. 2018. Studies with psychedelic drugs in human volunteers. *Neuropharmacology* 142(November):116–134. https://doi.org/10.1016/j.neuropharm.2017.11.029.

Shao, L.-X., C. Liao, I. Gregg, P. A. Davoudian, N. K. Savalia, K. Delagarza, and A. C. Kwan. 2021. Psilocybin induces rapid and persistent growth of dendritic spines in frontal cortex in vivo. *Neuron* 109(16):2535–2544. https://doi.org/10.1016/j.neuron.2021.06.008.

Vollenweider, F. X. 2001. Brain mechanisms of hallucinogens and entactogens. *Dialogues in Clinical Neuroscience* 3(4):265–279.

Vollenweider, F. X., and M. Kometer. 2010. The neurobiology of psychedelic drugs: Implications for the treatment of mood disorders. *Nature Reviews Neuroscience* 11(9):642–651. https://doi.org/10.1038/nrn2884.

Vollenweider, F. X., and K. H. Preller. 2020. Psychedelic drugs: Neurobiology and potential for treatment of psychiatric disorders. *Nature Reviews Neuroscience* 21(11):611–624. https://doi.org/10.1038/s41583-020-0367-2.

Wasson, R. G. 1957. Seeking the magic mushroom. *Life*, May 13, 1957.

Watts, R., and J. B. Luoma. 2020. The use of the psychological flexibility model to support psychedelic assisted therapy. *Journal of Contextual Behavioral Science* 15(January):92–102. https://doi.org/10.1016/j.jcbs.2019.12.004.

Zittoun, T., and S. Brinkmann. 2012. Learning as meaning making. In N. M. Seel (ed.), *Encyclopedia of the sciences of learning*. Boston, MA: Springer. https://doi.org/10.1007/978-1-4419-1428-6_1851.

B

Workshop Agenda

Exploring Psychedelics and Entactogens as
Treatments for Psychiatric Disorders

March 29–30, 2022

Statement of Task

A planning committee of the National Academies of Sciences, Engineering, and Medicine will organize and conduct a 1.5-day virtual public workshop that brings together experts and key stakeholders from academia, government, industry, and non-profit organizations to explore the use of psychedelics and entactogens—including LSD, psilocybin, and MDMA—as treatments for psychiatric disorders, such as major depressive disorder, anxiety disorder, posttraumatic stress disorder, and substance use disorders. Invited presentations and discussions will be designed to:

1. Review the current state of knowledge regarding the mechanisms of action and pharmacokinetic/pharmacodynamic properties of these compounds, including considering the impact of polypharmacy.
2. Discuss the current evidence on the clinical efficacy of psychedelics and entactogens to treat psychiatric conditions, including:
   a. exploring the role of adjunctive psychotherapy,
   b. discussing whether hallucinogenic and dissociative side effects are essential to treatment efficacy, and
   c. clarifying the importance of psychosocial contexts.

3. Consider the role of biomarkers to target treatments, stratify patients, and predict safety profiles.
4. Explore appropriate clinical trial design, the need for standardization of treatment regimens, the challenge of blinding and accounting for placebo effects, and regulatory considerations.
5. Discuss the impacts of these compounds' legal status and scheduling classifications on research.
6. Explore questions of biomedical ethics, such as those regarding pxatient protections and consent, standards of clinical training and quality assurance, off-label use, equitable access to treatment options, and engagement with public interest and experimentation.
7. Discuss open research questions, policy needs, and opportunities to move the field forward.

The planning committee will develop the agenda for the workshop, select and invite speakers and discussants, and moderate the discussions. A proceedings of the presentations and discussions at the workshop will be prepared by a designated rapporteur in accordance with institutional guidelines.

DAY 1, MARCH 29, 2022

9:30am
EST

Welcome and workshop overview, *10 min*
Sarah H. Lisanby, National Institute of Mental Health (NIMH), *Workshop Co-Chair*
Gerard Sanacora, Yale School of Medicine, *Workshop Co-Chair*

Session 1: An Introduction to Psychedelics and Entactogens as Treatments for Mental Health Conditions

Objectives:
1. Preview the key focus areas to be covered in the workshop.
2. Provide a high-level overview on the history of psychedelic medicine as treatments for mood and substance use disorders.
3. Highlight testimonials from individuals who can speak to the subjective experience of clinical treatment with these agents.

9:40am

Session overview, *5 min*
Moderator: Sarah H. Lisanby, NIMH, *Workshop Co-chair*

9:45am   Overview on the history of psychedelics and MDMA as treatments for psychiatric disorders, *15 min*
          Speaker: Charles Grob, University of California, Los Angeles (UCLA)

10:00am   **Personal perspectives on clinical treatment with psychedelics and MDMA,** *20 min*
          Speakers:
             Nora Osowski, MPH
             Lori Tipton, Psychedelic Society of New Orleans, Louisiana

10:20am   **Audience Q&A,** *5 min*

10:25am   **Break,** *10 min*

Session 2a: State of the Evidence on Mechanisms of Action and Key Research Gaps for Classic Psychedelics and MDMA

Objectives:
1. Review the state of knowledge regarding the acute and enduring molecular and circuit mechanisms of action, and the state of knowledge by which psychosocial contexts modulate those mechanisms.
2. Provide a summary from the January 2022 NIMH psychedelics workshop: What key research gaps were identified?

10:35am   **Session overview,** *5 min*
          Moderator: Rita Valentino, National Institute on Drug Abuse (NIDA)

10:40am   **Overview of the state of knowledge on molecular mechanisms of action,** *20 min*
          Speaker: Gabriella Gobbi, McGill University

11:00am   **Overview of the state of knowledge on circuit mechanisms of action,** *20 min*
          Speaker: Katrin Preller, Yale School of Medicine/University of Zurich

11:20am   **Overview of the state of knowledge on the neuroplastic effects,** *20 min*
          Invited speaker: David E. Olson, University of California, Davis

11:40am   **Overview of the state of knowledge on the role of psychosocial contexts,** *20 min*
Speaker: Rosalind Watts, Synthesis Institute

12:00pm   **Summary of research gaps identified in the January 2022 NIH psychedelics workshop,** *10 min*
Speaker: Nora Volkow, NIDA

12:10pm   **Audience Q&A,** *20 min*

12:30pm   **Lunch,** *1 hr*

Session 2b: Exploring Critical Research Gaps and Opportunities

Objectives:
1. Explore critical research gaps that need to be addressed to advance the field and discuss potential opportunities for action, including:
   a. What are the interactions between molecular/circuit mechanisms and the psychosocial context?
   b. During treatment, what other aspects of the patient's psychoemotional state are being modified (e.g., changes in beliefs, social bonding, consciousness, and spirituality), and what are the implications?
   c. Is the hallucinogenic/dissociative experience part of the therapeutic mechanism of action and what are the implications?

1:30pm   **Session overview:** John Krystal, Yale School of Medicine, *5 min*

1:35pm   **Panel discussion: Exploring three key research gaps,** *60 min*
Panelists:
Javier Gonzalez-Maéso, Virginia Commonwealth University
Roland Griffiths, Johns Hopkins University
Tristan McClure-Begley, Defense Advanced Research Projects Agency
Robert Malenka, Stanford University
Gitte Moos Knudsen, University of Copenhagen

2:35pm   **Audience Q&A,** *10 min*

2:45pm   **Break,** *10 min*

Session 3: Key Opportunities to Advance Clinical Development

Objectives:
1. Provide an overview of the current evidence of clinical efficacy of psychedelics and entactogens to treat mood and substance use disorders.
2. Discuss key regulatory considerations.
3. Explore two challenges/questions that are critical for moving this field forward, and discuss potential opportunities for action.

2:55pm   **Moderator introductions,** *5 min*
               Moderator: Gerard Sanacora, Yale School of Medicine, *Workshop Co-Chair*

3:00pm   **Landscape view of evidence of clinical efficacy,** *20 min*
               Invited speaker: Collin Reiff, New York University, Langone

3:20pm   **Key regulatory considerations,** *20 min*
               Speaker: Javier Muñiz, Food and Drug Administration (FDA)

3:40pm   **Break,** *5 min*

3:45pm   **Panel discussion: Major challenges for clinical development,** *60 min*
               1. How should clinical trial designs evaluate the impact of the non-pharmacological factors (e.g., guided treatment sessions [in-person versus digital administration; individual settings vs. group settings])
               2. How can clinical trial design address challenges related to blinding, active comparators, expectancy effects, and placebo effects?

               Panelists:
               Collin Reiff, New York University, Langone
               Javier Muñiz, FDA
               Luana Colloca, University of Maryland
               Srinivas Rao, atai Life Sciences
               Charles Raison, Usona Institute/University of Wisconsin–Madison
               Steven Levine, COMPASS Pathways
               Corine de Boer, Multidisciplinary Association for Psychedelic Studies Public Benefit Corporation

4:45pm   **Audience Q&A,** *10 min*

4:55pm   **Concluding remarks,** *5 min*
                Speakers: Gerard Sanacora, Yale School of Medicine, *Workshop Co-Chair*

5:00pm   **Adjourn**

DAY 2, MARCH 30, 2022

10:00am   **Welcome, recap of day 1 themes,** *10 min*
EST   Gerard Sanacora, Yale School of Medicine, *Workshop Co-Chair*

Session 4: Anticipating Implementation to Guide Clinical Research and Development

Objectives:
1. Identify anticipated implementation issues for psychedelic medicines and related treatments (should they be approved?), and discuss how these considerations should be used now to guide clinical development by exploring these discussion questions:
    a. How does the legal status of these agents shape the path to clinical implementation?
    b. What are the implications of possible abuse, misuse, and off-label use? Lessons learned from esketamine as a case study to compare with MDMA.
    c. What special bioethical and patient protection risks may arise during implementation (e.g., need to prevent the sexual abuse and exploitation of a patient's psychoemotional vulnerability), and how can risk mitigation approaches be studied during the rollout?

10:10am   **Session Overview,** *5 min*
                Moderator: Paul Appelbaum, Columbia University

10:15am   **Frameworks for accessible and equitable implementation,** *20 min*
                Speaker: Melissa A. Simon, Northwestern University

10:35am **Panel discussions: Critical challenges for implementation,** *70 min*
Panelists:
Melissa A. Simon, Northwestern University
Anthony Coulson, Drug Enforcement Administration
    (retired)/NTH Consulting, Inc.
Dominic Sisti, University of Pennsylvania
Charma D. Dudley, National Alliance on Mental Illness (NAMI)
Caroline Dorsen, Rutgers University School of Nursing
Steven Levine, COMPASS Pathways

11:45am **Audience Q&A,** *15 min*

12:00pm **Lunch,** *30 min*

Session 5: Synthesis and Next Steps

Objectives:
1. Synthesize key themes from the workshop.
2. Discuss critical research gaps, next steps, and promising opportunities for future action.

12:30pm **Session overview and synthesis of workshop's key themes,** *15 min*
Moderator: Sarah H. Lisanby, NIMH, *Workshop Co-Chair*

12:45pm **Panel discussion—Emerging themes and the road ahead,** *55 min*
Panelists:
Daniel Karlin, MindMed
Sean Belouin, Substance Abuse and Mental Health Services
    Administration, U.S. Public Health Service
Walter Dunn, UCLA
Shirley Holloway, NAMI
Joshua Gordon, NIMH
Nora Volkow, NIDA

1:40pm **Audience Q&A,** *15 min*

1:55pm **Concluding remarks,** *5 min*
Sarah H. Lisanby, NIMH, *Workshop Co-Chair*
Gerard Sanacora, Yale School of Medicine, *Workshop Co-Chair*

2:00pm **Adjourn**